Beat IBS

HILDA GLICKMAN

A How to Book

ROBINSON

ROBINSON

First published in 2016 by Robinson
1 3 5 7 9 10 8 6 4 2

Important Note
This book is not intended as a substitute for medical advice or treatment.
Any person with a condition requiring medical attention should consult a
qualified medical practitioner or suitable therapist.

A CIP catalogue record for this book is available from the British Library.

ISBN 978-1-47213-685-5

Typeset in Bembo by Initial Typesetting Services, Edinburgh
Printed and bound in Great Britain by Clays Ltd, St Ives plc

Papers used by Robinson are from well-managed forests and
other responsible sources.

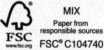

MIX
Paper from
responsible sources
FSC® C104740

Robinson
An imprint of
Little, Brown Book Group
Carmelite House
50 Victoria Embankment
London EC4Y 0DZ

An Hachette UK Company
www.hachette.co.uk

www.littlebrown.co.uk

How To Books are published by Robinson, an imprint of
Little, Brown Book Group. We welcome proposals from authors who
have first-hand experience of their subjects. Please set out the aims of
your book, its target market and its suggested contents in an email to
Nikki.Read@howtobooks.co.uk

This book is dedicated to my husband, Avrom,
who has helped and encouraged me throughout this
project and supports me in all that I do

CONTENTS

Contents

Contents

INTRODUCTION

Do you suffer from wind, bloating, constipation, diarrhoea or abdominal cramping? Have you been diagnosed with irritable bowel syndrome (IBS)? If so, you will know how distressing it can be. These symptoms are uncomfortable and embarrassing, upsetting and annoying, but I can assure you that you are not alone. IBS and other digestive problems are extremely common and affect a large percentage of the population at one time or other. The syndrome affects nearly 50 million people in the USA, while in the UK one-third of the population get IBS at some point in their lives.

You may have tried all sorts of remedies with little or limited success but I urge you not to lose heart. You *can* get better. IBS can be helped if you go about it the right way. The good news is that many people have used the programme in this book and solved their problems. Now you can too.

When I trained as a nutritionist, I learned how to help people with all sorts of health problems. However, it soon became clear that the bulk of my clients were coming to me with the same symptoms such as wind bloating, constipation and diarrhoea. In short, all sorts of digestive problems. Because

1

of this, I decided to concentrate mainly on those conditions and I found that people often improved very quickly.

It was so satisfying to see people, even those who had suffered for many years, get better. In fact, one person who had suffered from digestive problems for over forty years got better relatively easily on this programme. For others it took longer but they also became free of their symptoms and more comfortable, less bloated, more regular and more energetic.

Why other interventions don't work

Other interventions don't work because practitioners don't look for all possible causes. Sometimes they don't look for the cause at all, but just treat the symptoms. They may deal with one or two aspects such as food intolerance or low fibre, but many practitioners are not comprehensive enough. They often look for one simple answer. For example, your doctor might tell you to increase fibre, a natural therapist might test you for allergies and another might say you have a yeast overgrowth. Some sufferers might indeed have these, but you need to find out what is causing *your* problems. The nature of IBS means that in different people it can be caused by different things so you need to test for all possible causes in a systematic way, one at a time. This book will show you how to do this.

You need also to remember that your digestive system doesn't exist on its own: it is part of your whole body. If it is not functioning correctly you need to improve your health overall. This may seem a daunting task but do not be concerned: this book will show you how to do that too.

Why this plan works

- It looks for the underlying *cause/causes* of your problems. This is very important because it is vital to find out why you are suffering rather than just treating the symptoms.

- It is systematic. It checks through all possible causes in a logical order.

- It is comprehensive. It looks at everything that could be affecting you.

- It is specific to you. You may have similar symptoms to someone else but the causes may be different.

- It shows you how to test for them.

- It then shows you how to deal with them.

- It shows you how to eat as we should, resulting in an improvement in your overall health – the modern diet is not helpful for good digestion.

Searching for the cause

If you leave a tap on in the bathroom and water floods the room, you can do two different things. You can run around the room mopping up the water with lots of towels and flannels. That will work for a short time. Or you can turn off the tap for a permanent fix. Treating digestive problems can be a lot like this. If you have IBS, you can take laxatives for constipation, medication for wind or antacids for heart-burn but they won't cure the condition. If you do not find out why you are having these problems in the first place, they will keep returning. Just treating the symptoms is not enough.

Some IBS programmes such as the FODMAP diet (see also page 118) ask you to stop eating a whole range of foods. Many of these foods are highly nutritious and are needed in the diet. The point is that you *should* be able to digest most good natural foods like cabbage and broccoli, so you need to find out why you can't. It may be because you lack digestive enzymes or have a yeast overgrowth. This book can help you find the cause of your symptoms.

Many possible causes

IBS has many possible causes and you may have just one of these or more than one. For example, you may have a yeast overgrowth, you may have parasites or you may have both or neither. Alternatively, you may just be sensitive to a particular food. The aim of this book is to find out which cause is affecting you.

The good news is that often the problem can be treated quite easily and simply. Whatever the cause, this book can help you find it by testing for each in a systematic way. Very many of my clients have found relief by doing this so take heart that with some thought and consideration you can too!

Chapter 1

WHAT IS IBS?

Irritable bowel syndrome is not a disease, but rather a collection of symptoms. For example, you might go to the doctor complaining of gas, bloating, intermittent constipation, diarrhoea and abdominal pain. The doctor may then ask you to take various tests designed to rule out more serious conditions like coeliac disease, Crohn's disease or even bowel cancer. If these tests are negative, you are said to have IBS. This is called a 'diagnosis of exclusion', meaning that the doctor has excluded most other conditions. With these more serious problems, the digestive tract is abnormal in some way and its structure has changed. However, with IBS, it looks normal because there is nothing to see on a scan or from an internal test. It is not the structure of the digestive tract that has changed but the way it functions.

No tests can confirm that you definitely have IBS. It is called a 'syndrome' because it is a group of different symptoms rather than just one. If the doctor can find nothing wrong with your gut, you are told you have IBS and you may be given medications to help with some of the symptoms. Usually there is not time to look for all the possible underlying causes.

It is of course good that you do not have a more serious disease, and you can take comfort in this. However, the wind, bloating and other problems are still there and affecting your life so you need help to eradicate them. Although these symptoms are not the result of something serious, they are there for a reason and this underlying cause needs to be discovered so that you can do something about them. The aim of this book is to help you do just that.

IBS is very common

If you do have IBS, you are not alone. In fact, it is thought that most people have symptoms at some time in their lives, and it has also become much more prevalent in modern times. The problem is that most of us don't talk much about our bowel habits and are too embarrassed even to go to our doctor.

How is IBS diagnosed?

IBS has traditionally been a difficult thing for doctors to diagnose but an organisation in the United States, the Rome Foundation, has come up with the Rome III Criteria (2006), which makes it easier. According to this, the symptoms are:

- Recurrent abdominal pain or discomfort for some months with two or more of the following:
- improvement with defecation;
- onset associated with a change in frequency of stool;

- onset associated with a change in form (appearance) of stool.

The NICE criteria in the UK lists similar symptoms:

- Abdominal pain or discomfort;
- bloating;
- change in bowel habit.

IBS is often divided into different categories: IBS-C is where the main symptom is constipation and IBS-D is where the person suffers mainly from diarrhoea. Of course, this is just describing what the patient already knows so it doesn't take us very far.

As mentioned, one problem is that IBS can have the same symptoms as other more serious conditions so these need to be ruled out. One of these is inflammatory bowel disease (IBD), which means that there is something wrong, such as coeliac disease, with the bowel. It is important to be aware that any bleeding from the back passage should always be investigated so your doctor may ask for tests to rule out IBD.

Understanding the difference between IBS and IBD

If a patient has inflammatory bowel disease, they have something wrong with the structure of the digestive system itself and it will not look normal in diagnostic tests such as a colonoscopy. It will be damaged, as in the case of diverticular disease where the surface of the bowel becomes lined with pockets or pouches, or it might be inflamed as in the case of Crohn's disease. Another condition relating to damage is coeliac disease where the little hairs that line the intestines have eroded away. Unlike IBD, IBS is not about damage and there is no change in the intestines. It is just that the digestive system is not working as well as it should.

The role of functional medicine

Nutritional therapists and some doctors are now practising what is called functional medicine, where there is recognition that the same symptoms can have different causes. This is certainly true of IBS. Another idea in functional medicine is that the different parts of the body are not separate but are related. For example, skin problems like psoriasis can be caused by poor digestion and eczema can be caused by a lack of essential fats.

In addition to this, functional medical practitioners emphasize that diet and lifestyle affect our health dramatically. Often the cause of an illness relates to nutrition and environmental factors, and IBS is a condition that can easily be looked at in this way. Instead of just treating individual symptoms, such as giving an antacid for heartburn or a laxative for constipation, the idea is to find the *underlying cause* and deal with that. In the case of IBS, the same symptoms can have many different causes and the causes can be different in different people.

Finding out what is causing *your* IBS

One of the main purposes of this book is to find out what is causing *your* IBS, and we will be partners in that mission. I will show you how you can do this and you can then take steps to get rid of it. As outlined in the introduction, the aim of this book is to go through every cause in turn, help you assess whether that is a problem for you and, if so, explain how you can eradicate it.

We have said that IBS is not a disease but a collection of symptoms. It is not an illness in the same way that, for example, measles is an illness. With measles we know the cause, that it is a virus, and we know what is happening in the body and why. IBS is more like a headache in that it can have many causes and these can vary between different people.

The three main aims of this book

1. To help you find the cause of *your* symptoms.
2. To show you how to deal with the cause or causes.
3. To make your digestive system as healthy as it can be and improve your health overall.

This book is concerned with how well your digestive system is working. If you are experiencing problems such as IBS, constipation, diarrhoea, wind, bloating or abdominal discomfort then your digestive system is not functioning at its best. There are many possible reasons for this and the idea here is to find the cause that applies to you. This is done in a very organized, logical and structured way. It relates to what was called the 4R programme (involving removal, replacement, re-inoculation and repair, see Chapter 2), which was designed by Dr Jeffrey Bland and his associates at the Institute for Functional Medicine.

Before we begin

Before we begin you first need to see your GP to rule out any serious disease such as Crohn's disease, coeliac disease or cancer. If tests and scans do not reveal the cause of your problems, you now need to find out why your symptoms are there. If your digestion is not functioning as it should there has to be a good reason, and our aim is to find out what this is.

The good news

The symptoms of IBS can be very upsetting and annoying but the good news is that because there is nothing wrong with the structure of the digestive tract it can helped quite easily and quickly. Therefore, there are many reasons to feel heartened.

Chapter 2

THE FIVE-STEP PLAN

This programme works in a systematic way. The list below outlines the five steps you need to take to find out why you are having these problems and then deal with them, and Chapters 3 to 7 deal with each step in detail.

- *Step 1: Remove the bad*: Check for substances in your digestive tract that should not be there, then remove them, if needed.

- *Step 2: Replace the good*: Check for what you do need for good digestion but which you may lack. Replace this, if needed.

- *Step 3: Re-inoculate*: Increase the good bacteria that are needed in the digestive tract.

- *Step 4: Repair the digestive tract*: After these problems have been dealt with, heal any injury or inflammation.

- *Step 5: Eat well to protect* your digestive health forever.

Step 1: Removing what should not be in your digestive tract

The first thing you need to do to restore good digestion is to check for anything that might be in your system that should not be there. These are common causes of IBS so they need to be ruled out. The causes will vary depending on the person, and you may have only one of these or you may have two or three. The important thing is to find out which, if any, are affecting *you*. The usual culprits are:

- Small intestinal bacterial overgrowth (SIBO)
- Wheat-based foods
- Parasites
- Allergenic foods
- Candida

This book will help you find out if any of these factors are affecting you. Some can be tested simply at home, while other tests need to be arranged by your GP, but if any of the above appears to be a problem for you then this book will show you what to do about it. You can take heart in the knowledge that most of these causes are not very difficult to deal with. Some problems may need a change of diet and some may need supplements, while others may need medication for a short time. However, if you persevere, you should get there in the end.

Remember that there may be more than one thing going on at the same time. For example, you could have an overgrowth of yeast as well as parasites so you will need to deal with both. On the other hand, you might get better just by changing one aspect of your diet such as giving up wheat.

Step 2: Replacing what should be in your digestive tract

Having tested for SIBO, candida, etc. and dealt with any that affect you, you may have solved your problem. If not, the next step is to test for the things that you may lack and replace these, if needed. Even if you feel better already, it is a good idea to assess these too.

For good digestion, we need the following and, if we don't have enough, they can be replaced. As above, tests can be used to find out which of these apply to you.

- Stomach acid (hydrochloric acid)
- Digestive enzymes
- Fibre

In the following chapters, you will find home and other tests that can be carried out to see if you have enough of all of these. If not, they can be replaced with food or nutritional supplements for a short time. After all that has been done, you then need to replace the good bacteria that you have lost.

Step 3: Re-inoculating yourself with good bacteria

In our digestive system, we should have good amounts of beneficial bacteria. These do a wonderful job in helping us digest food and protect our health in many other ways. They include names like *Lactobacillus acidophilus* and *Bifidobacterium*. Together they are referred to as 'probiotics' and you will have seen many foods in the supermarket being promoted as containing these. There are many other beneficial bacteria and they are very important.

Unfortunately, many of us do not have enough good bacteria. One reason is that most of us were given antibiotics at some time in our lives for conditions such as tonsillitis and other infections. Unfortunately, these kill not just bad bacteria but some of our good bacteria as well. Good bacteria perform a wonderful job not just for digestion but also for health in general. Luckily, these can be replaced quite easily with foods and supplements. In this step we need to:

- replace the good bacteria first with supplements and then with foods;

- eat foods that help feed these good bacteria (prebiotics).

Step 4: Repairing your digestive tract

Once you have sorted out all of the above and your digestion is working more efficiently you then need to take steps to heal your digestive tract. If you have had these problems for a long time, you may have some minor damage or inflammation in the lining of your gut. The next step is to heal this with supplements, if needed, and the best anti-inflammatory foods.

Step 5: Eating the best diet for digestive health

Having been through all of the steps above your digestive system should now be functioning at its best. Chapter 7 will show you how to make sure that you keep your newfound digestive health in the long term by eating the right foods. These are the foods that nourish us the most and help prevent many illnesses and conditions. They are the foods that we have eaten and developed on for thousands of years and which we still need.

The overall programme

You can see that the five-step programme outlined here has a very logical structure. You may have been diagnosed with IBS or you may have just one problem such as constipation. You may just get a few symptoms from time to time or you may have constant difficulties. Either way, this programme is suitable for all. In fact, it can help most of us because no one's digestion is as good as it could be.

The programme you will find in the following pages should go a long way towards sorting out your individual problems and improving your digestion overall. On top of that, the suggestions for the healthiest way to eat should protect you from many other illnesses and health problems throughout your life.

We will go on this journey together. In the next chapter, we will take the first step and see whether a common bacterium is affecting *you*.

Chapter 3

REMOVING WHAT SHOULD NOT BE IN YOUR DIGESTIVE TRACT

You need to check for problems with the following and deal with them if need be:

- Small intestinal bacterial overgrowth (SIBO)
- Wheat-based foods
- Parasites
- Allergenic foods
- Candida.

Checking for small intestinal bacterial overgrowth (SIBO)

A good place to begin is to be tested for small intestinal bacterial overgrowth as research has shown that a large percentage of IBS sufferers have it. This test is not difficult as it is just a simple breath test. There appears to be an association between SIBO and IBS, and symptoms of SIBO are similar to other digestive problems.

One study published in the *Romanian Journal of Internal Medicine* found that 31 per cent of IBS patients tested also had SIBO.[1] Another piece of research supported this finding more dramatically, where a whopping 78 per cent of IBS of sufferers were found to have SIBO. In patients whose main symptom was diarrhoea, 45.7 per cent were found to have SIBO, underlining how important it is to be tested for this.

What is SIBO?

SIBO just means an overgrowth of bacteria in the small intestine. The small intestine connects your stomach to your colon or large intestine, and in pictures it looks like a large amount of wound-up tubing. It has to be wound up like this because it is not small at all: it's about seven metres in length (nearly as wide as a tennis court). The job of the small intestine is to break down and digest our food using enzymes produced by the pancreas. We can see the action of enzymes when we use washing-up liquid on greasy dishes. If you look carefully, you will see the large globules of fat breaking up and becoming smaller.

An important point about the small intestine is that it should not contain any bacteria as it is supposed to be sterile. While it is normal to have bacteria in the large intestine (or colon), it is not normal to have it in the small intestine. If bacteria (even good bacteria) find their way into that part of the body, problems can begin.

If bacteria do get in there they can cause symptoms like those of IBS because they eat our food and thrive on it. These annoying parasites act on any food that they can get hold of and the foods then start to ferment (see overleaf for the result). This happens particularly after eating sugars.

Symptoms of SIBO

- Bloating and gas especially after eating sugar, fibre or carbohydrates;

- abdominal pain;

- constipation;

- diarrhoea;

- sometimes frothy yellow stools.

You can see, therefore, that there is quite a similarity between symptoms of IBS and SIBO so it is a good idea to rule out the latter.

What causes SIBO?

Clinical nutritionist Elizabeth Lipski says that some people get SIBO because they do not have enough acid in their stomach.[2] The strong hydrochloric acid is supposed to kill all bad bacteria. If this is the case, how does SIBO occur? One reason is that sufferers of heartburn often feel they have too much acid and so take over-the-counter drugs to suppress it. Some of us even use proton pump inhibitors, which are given on prescription by the doctor. These do not just neutralize the acid, they actually stop us producing it. However, good levels of stomach acid are needed both to digest our food and to kill off any bugs that reach the stomach. Low stomach acid can allow bacteria, fungi and parasites to thrive and affect the digestive system further along.

Testing for SIBO

This is a simple test that involves swallowing a substance called lactulose or glucose and then collecting breath samples every twenty minutes for three hours. Although this test can apparently give some false positives it is still helpful. Your GP might do it or you can go to a private laboratory via a nutritionist.

Treatment of SIBO

The good news is that if you test positive for SIBO it can be easily treated with medication. The most common one is an antibiotic called Rifaximin, which you can get on prescription. Because this can have side effects, some natural health practitioners prefer to treat SIBO with substances such as garlic, grapefruit extract or oil of oregano. If you do take antibiotics, you should follow those with a good probiotic (beneficial bacteria) supplement to replenish your good bacteria. In any case, probiotics are sometimes given as a treatment in themselves. Retest after treatment to ensure that SIBO has gone.

Could wheat or gluten be causing *your* problems?

The trouble with wheat

Wheat is a very difficult substance to digest, so much so that practitioners often tell patients that they are intolerant to it. I am not going to tell you that because your digestion is not the problem here. The problem is the wheat itself. Wheat that we eat today is a bad food for most people because it is very difficult to digest and can damage the gut. Modern wheat is very different from the wheat that we ate in the past. It has been changed so dramatically that it is not found in nature and that is why so many people have a problem with it. Many of us experience great relief when we give it up.

Could wheat be causing *your* problems? This question is easy to answer. Just stop eating it for a few weeks to see how you feel. Of course, you would need to make sure that you are giving up wheat in all its forms and that means reading labels because wheat is found in many foods. You may feel worse for a few days as the wheat leaves your system but, after that, you could feel very much better than before.

Should you have a test for wheat intolerance? Not necessarily. You can be your *own* test. You will know if you feel better without it and you will know if you feel worse when adding it back into your diet. This really is the best test of all. However, if you want more proof, blood tests are available. These look for antibodies against wheat so you need to have the test before you stop eating it.

Are you a wheat junkie?

Do you love bread, cereals, cakes, biscuits and pasta? Do you feel a need to have these in the house at all times? I ask this because many of us do. Wheat-based foods are often eaten as soon as we rise and throughout the whole day in one form or another. Actually, we eat these foods more than any other type of food available.

Wheat comes in so many different varieties that it is extremely difficult to avoid and food manufacturers seem to be constantly dreaming up new ways to use it. Because it is so flexible, it turns up in masses of different foods in many interesting ways. It is amazingly versatile and can be twisted, puffed up, rolled and bent into all shapes and sizes, which is why it is included in so many different foods. It is found all over the supermarket, with long aisles of every type of bread under the sun to pastries, pies, cakes, biscuits, pasta and noodles. It is also contained in sauces, soups, breaded foods and ready meals, where it hides from the unsuspecting public.

Wheat, wheat, wheat: it has taken over our lives. If you think about it you will see that most people are actually living on it. For breakfast, they might have cereal, toast or both, or perhaps a croissant or pain au chocolate. Then they might have a biscuit at mid-morning, sandwiches for lunch, maybe a muffin or a Danish pastry with afternoon tea and some form of pasta dish for the evening meal. All of these are wheat. When I tell my clients this, they begin to see what a huge part wheat has come to play in their lives.

Wheat is easy money

In addition to that, have you noticed how many pizza and pasta restaurants have sprung up all over the place? These sell cheap food at quite a high price. Do you love going to coffee houses? Many of us do but if you want something to eat there the choices are mainly cakes, biscuits or sandwiches. When we are at the station or out and about it is not easy to find anything that is not made with wheat, apart from the odd (usually brown!) banana or chocolate. This is not doing us any good, whether we have IBS or not.

What is wrong with wheat, you might ask? Aren't we told to eat grains as part of a 'balanced diet'? They are sometimes called 'healthy whole grains'. This is a misnomer. They are not healthy at all. If you compare vegetables to these grains, vegetables win easily. They are far higher in nutrients, they are not allergenic; we have eaten them for all of our time on the planet; and, very importantly, they contain phytochemicals that help prevent cancer, heart disease and many other illnesses. On the other hand, wheat contains few of these and takes the place of more nutritious foods.

Why not wheat?

If you came to me for help the first thing that I would say to you is, 'Give up wheat.' As mentioned, this is not because I think you in particular are intolerant to it but simply because wheat itself is a bad food for most people. There are many reasons for this:

- Modern wheat is very difficult to digest.

- It contains high levels of gluten (see opposite).

- Eating it produces cravings for more.

- Most wheat-based foods contain few nutrients.

- It raises blood sugar higher than sugar itself.

- Wheat-based foods fill you up and take the place of more nutritious foods.

- Wheat has high levels of pesticides as it is an important crop financially.

- It contains opiate mimickers, which means you can become addicted to it.

- It has high levels of lectins (these are sticky substances that bind to the hairs that line the intestines and prevent them from working normally).

- As well as affecting our digestion, new evidence is coming in that wheat also affects our brain: neurologist David Perlmutter in his book *Grain Brain* argues that it is implicated in brain conditions such as Alzheimer's and dementia.[3]

- Because it can cause high levels of blood sugar, wheat contributes to obesity, diabetes and breast cancer.

- Excess sugar raises insulin and high levels of this are associated with breast cancer.

Wheat-free helps reduce IBS problems

Research shows that IBS and wheat are associated. For instance, a study in the *American Journal of Gastroenterology* has maintained that some patients 'with IBS symptoms respond symptomatically from the exclusion of gluten from the diet'.[4]

In my experience of the people who came to me, giving up wheat can have a dramatic effect on digestive problems including IBS. When I have asked clients to do this their wind and bloating went, their abdominal cramps often improved and they had more energy. An added bonus, which usually pleased them, was that they lost weight and inches, particularly from the tummy area.

I remember one client whose severe wind and abdominal pain cleared up when she gave up wheat and, when she ate it again, her pains came back. However, her friend told her that she should have a blood test to make sure that her problems really were caused by wheat. If she had a blood test and it came back negative, would she have continued eating wheat even if it made her feel ill? If you eat wheat and you're bloated and in pain, and you stop eating it and you're not bloated, what better test can there be? This type of exclusion test is the best test of all.

Wheat affects most of us

Very many people have trouble with wheat and it could still be affecting them even if they do not have obvious symptoms. If you are having digestive problems there is a good chance that modern wheat is not helping. I say 'modern wheat' because it wasn't always like this. You might think that we have been eating wheat since time began but this is not so. While we have been on the planet for around 2.6 million years, wheat was introduced only in the last 10,000 years, just a moment in terms of our evolution.

In addition to this, the modern grains bear little resemblance to the grains we ate even twenty years ago, which is a problem. Our modern wheat is not as Mother Nature intended but something dreamed up by scientists in a laboratory.

How has wheat changed?

Wheat became a different food at the end of the twentieth century. The changes were made mainly for financial gain through increasing yield and decreasing the cost of production. They were not made to make it more nutritious or to help the consumer. Unfortunately, little thought was given to whether it would be good for us and no one worried about it being easy to digest. We now know that it is neither. New strains have been developed by cross breeding and mating with other strains and grasses, and this has led to a product humankind had never seen before. As Dr William Davis put it, 'Wheat gluten proteins, in particular, undergo considerable structural change with hybridization. In one hybridization experiment, fourteen new gluten proteins were identified in the offspring that were not present in either wheat plant'.[5] Although this gave much higher yields and farmers were happy, we do not really know how these affect our health.

Davis makes the point that because this came about before the advent of testing for safety it escaped the procedures that are in place today. He says that it occurred at a time when no questions were asked. He argues that 'the genetic variations introduced with each round of hybridization can make a world of difference'. And with wheat, there are thousands of hybridizations. No wonder modern wheat can cause such problems.

Foods that are mainly wheat	
bread	paninis
bagels	pasta
biscuits	pies
breadcrumbs	pitta
breakfast cereals	pizza
cakes	poppadums
couscous	pretzels
crackers	rolls
croissants	rusks
croutons	samosas
crumpets	sausage rolls
doughnuts	scones
gravy	tabbouleh
matzos	waffles
noodles	wheat bran
pain au chocolate	wraps
pancakes	

So many foods contain wheat that it is no wonder our digestions are not what they should be. It is amazing how creative we have been with this one food, a food that is relatively new to our diet.

On top of this, there is hidden wheat everywhere. Manufacturers put wheat or gluten into many foods that you might not suspect, including soups, stews, sauces, ready meals, nutritional supplements, soy products and more. This means that we are getting a constant injection of wheat throughout the whole day, every day.

We do not need wheat

You may have heard that wheat is a food group and be told that if you give it up you will be missing something important. This is not true. White flour contains very few nutrients and just acts as a filler. All the nutrients are contained in the germ of the wheat, which is discarded when the flour is processed. This goes for wheat made into bread, cakes and pasta. Whole-wheat flour does contain the germ but it is still not an important food because you can get all the nutrients you need from other, better foods. The fact that it has been called a food group is just arbitrary as there is no good reason for this. As mentioned earlier, we have lived without wheat for most of our time on this planet so we do not need it now.

Is wheat addictive?

Do you have a craving for wheat? I like it myself, I must admit, and there is no doubt that many people do. They feel better after eating it and feel a need to have it regularly, but they eat it so often that they do not realize this is happening. Do you come down in the morning and immediately reach for the toaster or bread bin? Or do you creep down in the middle of the night to have some cereal and milk? If you do, you are certainly not alone.

You may think that addiction is an odd word to use when talking about bread, but we now know that chemicals in wheat called polypeptides can cross the blood/brain barrier. This barrier is there to prevent certain substances getting to the brain, but wheat molecules can cross this. They attach themselves to the brain's morphine receptors and produce a kind of high. Dr Christine Zioudrou called them 'exorphins', as they are similar to the endorphins that we produce in our own bodies.[6] They give us a lift and make us feel good, but this does not mean wheat is doing us good.

Wheat's addictive quality means we are drawn to it like a moth to a flame and we often feel bad if we don't have it. Does this sound like withdrawal symptoms? That is exactly what it is. This is what keeps us returning to wheat-based foods again and again and makes us shudder with horror when asked to give it up. When I began to give up bread I noticed that I kept looking wistfully at pasta in the supermarket. As I never eat pasta, I wondered why and then I realized that I was craving wheat. This is because the gluten in wheat contains drug-like chemicals called gluteomorphins. They bid to opiate receptors in the brain, which makes us crave them more and more.

What is gluten?

This is the part of wheat that gets the most publicity, and it is also found at lower levels in other grains like oats and barley. Gluten is well known because it causes coeliac disease (see Chapter 8), a condition where the villi or small hairs in the intestines are destroyed or flattened. These hairs are very important because they help us absorb our food by increasing the surface area. However, for now we are looking at the problem of gluten for those who have IBS but not coeliac disease. This is so common nowadays that it has now been given its own name: *non-coeliac gluten sensitivity*. Although most people do not have coeliac disease, any food that can do what gluten does to the villi must really be suspect for us all.

Gluten acts like glue

The word 'gluten' comes from the Latin word for 'glue'. It is not difficult to see why. Parents sometimes make sticky paste for their children with flour and water, which sticks because the flour contains the gluey gluten. It is used in baking breads because it makes the dough elastic and helps it to rise and keep its shape, and it also makes pasta chewy and croissants fluffy. No other grain can perform these feats so it is no wonder that the food industry just loves it. The problem is that your digestive system probably doesn't.

I am often asked about wholemeal bread as this is promoted as being better than white bread. In some ways it is, as it contains the germ of the wheat with all its nutrients, but wholemeal bread contains even more gluten. Wholemeal dough is heavier and bakers have trouble making it rise so they add extra gluten, which is good for the baker but not the consumer!

Gluten and IBS

Gluten grains should be avoided by those with IBS. One study published in the journal *Nutrients* stated that, 'several studies have shown that a large number of patients who are fulfilling the criteria for irritable bowel syndrome IBS are sensitive to gluten'.[7] They carried out a trial where the patients were divided into two groups and given different diets. The results showed that a large number of the patients with IBS were actually sensitive to gluten. This does not surprise me. In fact, Dr William Davis calls IBS, 'coeliac disease lite', a very interesting description![8] He makes the point that when wheat is removed from the diet IBS improves.

Gluten has been changed dramatically in the last forty years or so. It is now harder to digest as the number of chromosomes it contains has changed. Gluten is a protein but unlike most proteins, which have a straight shape that allows them to be broken down by digestive enzymes, it is shaped like a spiral, making it more difficult to break down.

Gluten is just the beginning

Gluten may be a big problem but there are other parts of wheat that are bad for us. According to Davis, there are over a thousand other proteins in wheat that can affect us.

Wheat substitutes

Wheat substitutes have been produced because so many of us cannot digest wheat properly. There are breads, pastas, pittas, biscuits and cakes made from other flours such as rice flour or potato flour. I am not particularly keen on these because they are highly processed and not particularly nutritious. However, for a special occasion or an odd time they can be used and at least they do not contain gluten. Rice cakes are better. They are not particularly nutritious either, but contain few artificial additives and are less processed. They are fine as a base for toppings like chopped herring, hummus or nut butters, which are difficult to eat on their own. For carbohydrate, it is better to eat potatoes and other starchy vegetables like carrots, swede and sweet potatoes rather than wheat substitutes. In food charts, we often forget that these are actually carbohydrate foods and they are often just labelled as vegetables.

Wheat-free, gluten-free breakfasts

Many people can face doing without wheat at dinner but wheat-free breakfasts are a challenge for some. We are so used to having cereals and toast that many children think that breakfast *means* cereals. However, it wasn't always the case. Where would our wheat have come from in times gone by before we began to cultivate it?

Bread and cereals are quick and easy to prepare but see below for a list of other easy foods that will nourish you much better. Breakfast can be any healthy food that you like as long as it doesn't cause blood sugar levels to drop too low later in the day. To keep blood sugar stable you should have some protein such as leftover chicken, fish, egg, tofu, cottage cheese, yogurt, etc. with some complex carbohydrate such as vegetables, brown rice or gluten-free bread, plus two teaspoons olive oil or some seeds or a little butter.

Breakfast ideas

- Porridge, egg, banana.
- Leftover soup with lots of vegetables.
- Leftover organic chicken salad mixed with brown rice, apple.
- Fish (not smoked), any vegetables except tomatoes, rice cakes, butter.
- Organic meat hamburger, gluten-free bread, banana
- Salmon (try to get organic fresh salmon, wild rather than farmed) on rice cakes, banana.

- Millet, well-cooked until soft with grated goat's cheese, mashed banana.
- Tinned sardines in brine (wash off brine), rice, little butter, half banana.
- Quinoa (similar to couscous, available from health-food shops) with carrots, goat's milk yogurt.
- Kedgeree (soft, well-cooked brown rice mixed with flaked white fish, peas, tomatoes).
- Natural rice crispies from health-food shops, goat's milk.
- Gluten-free bread with egg or tinned fish (wash off oil or brine).

Checking for parasites

The thought of having strange organisms in your digestive tract might make you shudder. However, these are becoming very common because we are travelling so much more than previously. Often when we go abroad we get a tummy bug but it gets better and we think no more about it. Unfortunately, some of these can linger and cause all sorts of problems later on. Some of the symptoms of parasites are constipation, bloating, gas, abdominal cramping, muscle aches and, strangely enough, teeth grinding and insomnia.

Parasites and IBS

One study found that 49 per cent of people with IBS had the parasite *Blastocystis hominis* and 20 per cent had the parasite *Dientamoeba fragilis*. This is known to cause IBS-type symptoms. You can be tested for these parasites on the NHS but some argue that some private laboratories are better able to find them. A review of studies in *The International Journal of Parasitology* concluded that, 'It is essential that all patients with IBS undergo routine parasitology investigations in order to rule out the presence of protozoan parasites as the causative agents of the clinical signs.'[9]

If you do have parasites, they can be dealt with either using medication from your doctor or herbal remedies.

Common parasites

- *Blastocystis hominis*
- *Giardia*
- *Dientamoeba fragilis*
- Pinworms.

Tests for parasites

As the parasites lurk in your system, the test involves a stool sample. In the UK, you can be tested on the NHS but some private laboratories may have better testing facilities, and you should go to one that specializes in testing for parasites. The company Genova Diagnostics (www.gdx.net) does a comprehensive parasitology screening as well as other stool tests. It might be a good idea to seek the advice of a qualified nutritional therapist (making sure that, in the UK, they are a member of the British Association for Applied Nutrition and Nutritional Therapy [BANT]).

If you do have parasites, they can be eradicated with medication or natural supplements. However, even if you do not have parasites now it is a good idea to take care to prevent getting them in the future (see the box below).

Treating parasites

Your doctor can help you with this. If you take medication to remove the parasites, you should re-inoculate the gut with probiotics afterwards, and you should retest after treatment to make sure that the parasites have gone. Natural remedies take about a month to be effective. These are:

- garlic;

- goldenseal or berberine;

- black walnut;

- wormwood;

- grapefruit seed extract.

Parasite prevention

It is a good idea always to take steps to prevent getting parasites in the future.

- Drink filtered or even boiled water.

- Eat organic food not sprayed with pesticides, but wash it thoroughly.

- Cook food above the minimum temperature to kill parasites (and bacteria), which is 180°F (82°C), but cook meat at 325°F (163°C) or higher and bake fish at 400°F (204°C), 8–10 minutes per inch of thickness.

- Beware of, or avoid raw foods such as sushi (Japan, China and Korea have a high incidence of infection from raw fish).

- Sanitize all toilet seats and bowls particularly those used by children.

- Don't walk barefoot, especially in warm, moist, sandy soil.

- Don't use tap water to clean contact lenses. Use sterilized lens solution.

- Keep toddlers away from puppies and kittens that have not been regularly dewormed, and don't let them kiss animals.

- Don't eat salads and uncooked food in non-Western countries.

- At parties or in pubs don't eat nuts or crisps from communal bowls. Buy your own and eat them yourself!

- It's best to avoid microwaving meats, as many microwaves do not cook evenly.

Allergenic foods: Do you have a food intolerance or allergy?

Have you ever wondered if you might be allergic or intolerant to certain foods? Nowadays more and more people seem to feel that they cannot tolerate one thing or another, but others argue that food allergies are not common. Who is right?

The problem is that there are different types of sensitivity to food. We often hear about food allergies and food intolerance, but what is the difference? The answer is that a true food allergy is something that affects us immediately after eating. For example, some people can become very ill after eating shellfish or certain nuts; the response is quick and the situation can become serious and may include anaphylactic shock. This should be treated as an emergency.

Food allergies are usually related to certain specific foods. The most common allergens are cow's milk, egg, peanuts, tree nuts, soya and shellfish. Children can be allergic to these foods more so than adults. According to the NHS, 'true' allergies affect just 2 per cent of the population and 8 per cent of children under the age of three. This type of true allergic reaction is called an immunoglobulin E (IgE) allergy because IgE antibodies are produced in the blood when the offending food is eaten. If you suspect that you have this type of allergy you should ask your doctor about it.

The charity Allergy UK confirms that 45 per cent of the population appear to be intolerant to some foods. There are different sorts of tests for possible food intolerance, some of which involve looking at blood samples. In one study where people were given an allergy-free diet for a year, a very large number improved and 88 per cent were relieved of bloating. There are various private laboratories in the UK that can test you for food allergies.

Food intolerance

This is different from a food allergy in many ways. Food intolerance is much more common and more difficult to diagnose because we can react to many different foods and often we eat these together. With food intolerance, the reaction will be less severe and the symptoms will be different. It can also show itself up to forty-eight hours after eating the food. This type of sensitivity is called an immunoglobulin G (IgG) reaction because the body makes IgG antibodies when in contact with the food.

Reactions are likely to be bloating, stomach cramps, rashes or fatigue. Food intolerance can be detected in blood tests but often the best test is to exclude the foods that most commonly cause intolerance and add them back one at a time.

Do you crave certain foods?

Strangely enough, the foods that you really crave and eat often affect you the most. Are there any foods that you just have to eat every day? Wheat and dairy certainly come into this category for many people. The thought of giving them up can make us feel very uneasy. We eat them all the time so we never really have withdrawal symptoms. As soon as we get the craving we just eat another piece of bread or another biscuit, and we tend to go for these foods when we are tired or upset or late at night. We do not realize that wheat or dairy are affecting us at all.

Sometimes when I have advised clients to give up certain foods they look horrified and say that if they did there would be nothing left to eat. This is a clear sign that they are craving these foods and that these foods are forming the major part of their diets. Some foods can actually be addictive: we feel better after eating them but want them again a few hours later.

The tomato: Just one example

Although wheat and dairy are the most obvious suspects, some people react to unexpected foods. Do you love tomatoes? I must admit I do and I can eat them in any form. I know of people who need to have tomatoes every day, and they feel uncomfortable if they do not have some ready to hand in the fridge. However, tomatoes really can be a problem for some people. They are part of the nightshade family (along with potatoes, aubergines and peppers), and can promote inflammation in the body affecting conditions like arthritis.

An interesting point is that three of the most common allergenic foods, wheat, dairy and tomatoes, are very often eaten together in certain foods. These include pizzas, lasagne, spaghetti bolognaise, other pasta dishes, cheese and tomato sandwiches or minestrone soup with cheese on the top. It is amazing that so many readymade meals sold in supermarkets contain tomatoes and wheat or wheat and cheese or even all three, and that so many of the recipes we use at home are the same.

Tomatoes, of course, may not be a problem for you. I have included them to show that an ordinary food that is considered generally good can be a problem for some people.

The elimination and challenge diet: The sensitive seven

In this type of home test, you cut out the most common allergenic foods. Then you reintroduce them one at a time and see how you feel. This diet is not too drastic and can even be quite pleasant, but it does cut out some foods that you might be craving. After a few days, on the other hand, you should begin to feel much more comfortable. You might even find that you begin to lose weight on the diet, which is an added bonus for many people! The foods below are often the most troublesome:

- Wheat
- Dairy (including all forms such as milk, cheese, yogurt, sheep's and goat's milk)
- Eggs
- Soya

- Tomatoes
- Peanuts
- Citrus fruits

The idea is that you cut out these foods for a few weeks and then introduce them back one at a time and watch your reaction. Remember that when it comes to food intolerance rather than food allergies, the unpleasant symptoms may not happen until up to forty-eight hours after eating. Therefore, you need to wait for a few days before introducing another food. This method is quite time consuming but it is really the best way to find out which foods could be affecting you. The two worst offenders seem to be wheat and dairy.

Can you digest dairy foods?

Many people have difficulty digesting dairy foods. Intolerance to dairy is quite a common problem and, in some societies, it is not consumed at all. If this is a problem for you, it will result in bloating, abdominal discomfort and diarrhoea. To rule it out, see the tests below.

Some may not be able to cope with the protein in milk, which is called casein, and others cannot digest the sugar in milk, called lactose. The latter have this problem because they lack in the enzyme lactase. This is not really intolerance as such as it just means that you cannot produce enough of this important enzyme to be able to digest milk sugar. Lactose intolerance is more likely where diarrhoea is the main symptom of the IBS sufferer. It is found in most dairy products but hard cheeses and butter have very low levels.

Some nationalities are more likely than others to have this problem. Apparently 90 per cent of Asians and 75 per cent of Africans are affected, but only around 15 per cent of Caucasians.

Testing for allergies and intolerances

Tests for food allergies

- *Blood test*: The blood test for IgE antibodies involves sending a sample of your blood to a laboratory through your doctor or allergy clinic. Private labs also do this test.

- *Pinprick test*: You can get a pinprick test from the doctor or hospital.

- *Elimination diet*: A much cheaper way of testing is simply to eat a diet that eliminates the most common allergenic foods, reintroducing them one at a time. However, if the possible allergic reaction is serious, you should seek medical advice before reintroducing foods.

Tests for food intolerance

- *Blood test*: This is for IgG antibodies, usually carried out in private laboratories.

- *Elimination diet*: This is where you eliminate the foods most commonly associated with intolerance and assess how you feel. Despite what a blood test might find, actually eating or not eating these foods shows you how they really do affect you.

Test for lactose intolerance

To find out if you cannot digest lactose you can have a hydrogen breath test via your doctor. You fast for twelve hours and then blow into a balloon to see how much hydrogen is present. You then have a drink that contains lactose and your breath is tested again over the next few hours. If the level of hydrogen has gone up, this shows that you are not digesting the lactose properly.

Candida: You may have an overgrowth of yeast

Are you all blown up?

Have you ever made bread using yeast? If so, you will know that if you place yeast together with sugar it becomes all frothy and bubbly, and this makes the bread rise. If we have yeast in our digestive system it can also cause lots of bubbling in our gut. This is what really does happen. If you are having trouble with wind, bloating, constipation and other digestive problems, you could have an overgrowth of yeast. It can make us feel like we have put on many pounds.

However, we are not talking here about baker's yeast. We are talking about *Candida albicans* (referred to as candida), a yeast that is more and more commonly making its home in our intestines. Most of us have it to some extent but, unless it becomes overgrown, it usually stays around doing little harm.

Yeast travels all over

An overgrowth of yeast in the digestive tract can make us feel very bloated and uncomfortable indeed, like our stomach has blown up like a balloon. That is not all it does. It can change from a yeast to a fungus and this allows it to burrow through the gut wall. If it does, it has access to our bloodstream and can then travel all over the body, creating problems and causing annoying symptoms anywhere.

If it sits on the tongue, you can see it as a thick white or yellow coating. In women, it can also manifest itself as a discharge that looks like cottage cheese. In these places, it tends to be called thrush. Fortunately, it can be removed easily with anti-fungal lozenges or suppositories. However, when it moves further, it can also cause other irritating problems like athlete's foot, fungal toenails, skin rashes and all the symptoms listed in the questionnaire on page 49. It is not exactly dangerous but it can make our lives very difficult if it takes hold. However, for now we are looking at candida in the digestive tract.

The good news is that if yeast overgrowth is your problem you need not worry because it is quite easy to deal with. We never really get rid of it completely but it is possible to reduce it enough to make you feel very much better. This can happen quite quickly if it is treated properly.

Candida is still with us

In the past looking for candida was very popular and it was blamed for all sorts of conditions. Consequently, some doctors thought that those in the alternative health sector were over-diagnosing it and blaming it for just about everything. This happens much less so today. Nowadays we seem to hear much less about it. However, this does not mean that it has gone away. It is just that fashions in healthcare change.

Perhaps in the past too much attention *was* paid to it, but now it might be under-diagnosed. It has not gone away. In fact, with the large amount of sugar that is eaten nowadays it is probably very much still here, causing as many digestive problems as it did before. It needs to be ruled out if someone is suffering from wind and bloating. If this annoying little parasite is the cause of *your* digestive problems, the good news is that when yeast is treated, people feel so much better and other complaints such as eczema or weight gain can improve as a side benefit.

Where does candida come from?

An overgrowth of candida can be caused by many things, including the overuse of antibiotics. Although these have been a great boon to humankind, many doctors would agree that they have been overused. Often patients demand them for every little sniffle. However, we now know that they work only on bacteria and not viruses.

The problem is that unfortunately, antibiotics are not too particular in their choice of bacteria. While they are very effective in killing off the nasty bacteria that give us infections like tonsillitis, they are also able to kill off the good bacteria that we need. These bacteria are there to fight off other harmful microbes and yeasts so killing them off leaves room for candida to grow and proliferate. Doctors know this and often find that women given antibiotics come back later suffering from thrush. To stop this happening in the past beneficial bacteria or probiotics were routinely given to patients on antibiotics, but now patients are usually left to buy their own.

Antibiotics are not just given to humans. Animals are dosed with them too. They are given routinely to prevent infections even when they are not ill and, unfortunately, they can stay on the meat. This is one good reason why organic meat is better: organic farmers are not permitted to use antibiotics except for genuine illness.

Candida loves sugar

An overgrowth of candida also results from our great love of sugar. We love it and eat far more of it than we used to. Unfortunately, yeast loves it too. As mentioned, if you make bread, you put the yeast in with the sugar so that it grows and all bubbles up but, if there is no sugar, the yeast dies. Having candida in itself makes us crave sugar and the more we eat, the more it grows.

As well as sugar and antibiotics, other things that encourage candida to grow are birth-control pills, hormone replacement therapy, chronic stress (because this causes more sugar to enter our bloodstream) and the use of steroid medications. Sometimes it becomes worse in women before a period or when pregnant as the hormones oestrogen and progesterone can affect it.

Is candida your problem?

The most common digestive symptoms of yeast overgrowth are constipation, bloating, diarrhoea, tiredness, mood swings, PMT and recurring vaginal or bladder infections. Strangely enough, sensitivities to perfumes or other strong odours are another symptom. As mentioned, candida can affect the whole body if it gets into the bloodstream. This can cause foggy thinking, muscle aches, anxiety and depression, and all of the symptoms listed in the questionnaire on page 49. It can also damage the lining of the small intestine, causing it to become permeable or 'leaky'.

Tests for candida

Various different tests can be carried out to check for candida. Some are simple home tests, some are questionnaires and others are tests that can be carried out by private laboratories. It might be a good idea to start with the simplest first and go on from there. Try the saliva test and then answer the questionnaires. These are not foolproof but give a good indication that candida might be your problem. Remember that we all have some candida in our systems so some tests like the saliva test may be positive regardless. We are looking here for an *overgrowth* of the yeast.

- *Saliva home test*: This is a simple home test for the presence of candida. It is not clear how reliable it is but it might be a good place to start, so treat it as an indication rather than proof. Place a glass of water beside your bed at night. When you wake up, before eating or brushing your teeth, spit into the water. After a while look to see if the spit forms vertical lines that descend from the top down. If present, this gives an indication of candida.

- *Saliva laboratory test*: This is a saliva test that is sent to a laboratory via a nutritionist.

- *Organic acid test*: One practitioner that I respect thinks that this is the best test for detecting an overgrowth of candida. The test is useful because it also shows whether we are metabolizing fatty acids properly. It also looks for low vitamin B levels, inflammatory reactions and more. For this test you send a urine sample to a laboratory for analysis (a nutritionist can arrange this for you).

- *Candida antibodies test*: This can be done by taking your blood at home using a pinprick and sending it off to a laboratory. There is also a saliva test for these. This test tells you if you have candida and the stage at which it is at.

- *Questionnaires*: The other home 'test' that you can do is to complete the questionnaires below. This does not give actual proof but, in conjunction with test results, it gives a good indication of a candida overgrowth.

Candida albicans *questionnaire*

SECTION 1: HISTORY

Add together the points for the questions to which the answer is 'Yes' and enter the score at the bottom of the table.

	Score
1. Have you taken Tetracyclines such as Sumycin and Panmycin or other antibiotics for one month or longer?	35
2. Have you ever taken broad-spectrum antibiotics for respiratory, urinary or other infections for two months or longer?	35
3. Have you taken a broad-spectrum antibiotic, even for a single course?	6
4. Have you ever been bothered by persistent prostatitis, vaginitis or other problems affecting your reproductive organs?	25
5. Have you been pregnant two or more times?	5
a. Have you been pregnant once?	3
6. Have you taken birth control pills for more than two years?	15
a. Have you taken the above for six months to two years?	8

7. Have you taken prednisone, Decadron or other cortisone-type drugs for more than two weeks?	15
a. Have you taken the above for two weeks or less?	6
8. Does exposure to perfumes, insecticides, fabric shop odours and other chemicals provoke severe/moderate symptoms?	20
a. Does exposure to the above provoke mild symptoms?	5
9. Are symptoms worse on mild, muggy days or in mouldy places?	20
10. Have you had severe or persistent athlete's foot, ringworm, 'jock itch' or other chronic fungal infections of the skin or nails?	20
a. Have you had any of the above mildly/moderately?	10
11. Do you crave sugar?	10
12. Do you crave breads?	10
13. Do you crave alcohol?	10
14. Does tobacco smoke *really* bother you?	10

Total score Section 1: . . . . . .

SECTION 2: MAJOR SYMPTOMS

Enter the appropriate figure in the point score column.

If a symptom is occasional or mild: 3 points

If a symptom is frequent and/or moderately severe: 6 points

If a symptom is severe and/or disabling: 9 points

Enter the total score at the end of the table.

	Score
1. Fatigue or lethargy	
2. Feeling of being 'drained'	
3. Depression	
4. Poor memory	
5. Feeling 'spacey' or 'unreal'	
6. Inability to make decisions	
7. Numbness, burning or tingling	
8. Headache/migraine	
9. Muscle aches	
10. Muscle weakness or paralysis	

11. Pain and/or swelling in joints	
12. Abdominal pain	
13. Constipation and/or diarrhoea	
14. Bloating, belching or intestinal gas	
15. Vaginal burning, itching or discharge	
16. Prostatitis	
17. Impotence	
18. Loss of sexual desire or feeling	
19. Endometriosis or infertility	
20. Cramps and/or menstrual irregularities	
21. Premenstrual tension	
22. Attacks of anxiety or crying	
23. Cold hands or feet and/or chilliness	
24. Shaking or irritable when hungry	

Total score Section 2: . . . . . .

SECTION 3: OTHER SYMPTOMS

For each of your symptoms, enter the appropriate figures in the point score column:

Symptom occasional or mild: 1 point

Symptom frequent and/or moderately severe: 2 points

Symptom severe and/or disabling: 3 points

Please note: While the symptoms in this section commonly occur in people with a yeast-connected illness, they are also found in other individuals. There are many causes for the symptoms outlined but the questionnaire combined with the tests described above can give a good indication of whether or not candida is a problem for you.

	Score
1. Drowsiness	
2. Irritability or jitteriness	
3. Lack of coordination	
4. Inability to concentrate	
5. Frequent mood swings	
6. Insomnia	
7. Dizziness/loss of balance	

8. Pressure above ears/feeling of head swelling	
9. Tendency to bruise easily	
10. Chronic rashes or itching	
11. Numbness, tingling	
12. Indigestion or heartburn	
13. Food sensitivity or intolerance	
14. Mucous in stools	
15. Rectal itching	
16. Dry mouth or throat	
17. Bad breath	
18. Foot, hair or body odour not relieved by washing	
19. Nasal congestion or postnasal drip	
20. Nasal itching	
21. Sore throat	
22. Laryngitis, loss of voice	
23. Cough or recurrent bronchitis	
24. Pain or tightness in chest	

25. Wheezing or shortness of breath	
26. Urinary frequency or urgency	
27. Burning or urination	
28. Spots in front of eyes or erratic vision	
29. Burning or tearing of eyes	
30. Recurrent ear infections or fluid in ears	
31. Ear pain or deafness	
32. Rash or blisters in mouth	

Total score Section 3: . . . . . .

RESULTS

Total score Section 1: . . . . . .

Total score Section 2: . . . . . .

Total score Section 3: . . . . . .

Overall score: . . . . . .

NB Scores in women will be higher as there are more questions that apply to them.

ANALYSING THE RESULTS

Scores of over 180 for women, over 140 for men: Yeast-connected health problems almost certainly present.

Scores of over 120 in women and over 90 in men: Yeast-connected health problems are probably present.

Scores of over 60 in women and over 40 in men: Yeast-connected health problems are possibly present.

(Taken from Crook, 1988)[10]

How to deal with candida

To kill off candida you need to starve it of its food supply and that means sugar. To get rid of it you need to stop eating sugar as well as foods that convert to sugar very quickly. These are refined carbohydrates like white bread, other white flour products and pasta. Of course, there is some sugar in vegetables but we need these and they do not cause spikes in blood sugar the way processed foods do. Although we need to cut off the yeast's food supply as much as possible by avoiding sugar, we do have to eat well. So do not be alarmed. It is possible to devise a pleasant, nutritious diet that allows us to stop feeding the yeast and still be satisfied (see overleaf for the anti-candida diet).

After about a month, you can then begin to take natural anti-fungal supplements. (Another route is to ask your doctor for medical anti-fungals like nystatin but it is gentler to go down the natural route and use nutritional supplements.)

The reason for trying to kill off the yeast slowly is that if too much is killed off too quickly you can begin to feel unwell. This is because dead candida produces toxins, which will disappear as you excrete them through your bowel movements.

The diet is quite restrictive but aside from not eating sugar, which is not good anyway, you do not need to be on it forever. As candida can mimic or lead to all sorts of other conditions, you may be surprised that other problems may clear up while on this diet. For example, one of my clients saw her eczema completely disappear and psoriasis is another skin complaint that is related to candida.

The anti-candida diet

This should be taken for the first month and then the anti-candida supplements can be added to the diet.

AVOID:

- Sugar in any form and all food containing sugar: including white, brown and castor sugar, honey, glucose, molasses, malt, syrup, fructose, cakes, biscuits, ketchup, ice cream, soft drinks, desserts and fruit juice (check labels as sugar can be found in unlikely foods such as peas, soups and ready meals).

- Yeast: including bread, food in breadcrumbs, Marmite, Bovril, citric acid, monosodium glutamate and vitamin tablets not labelled 'yeast free'.

- Refined grains: including white flour, granary flour, white rice, white pasta, cornflour, custard powder, cornflakes and cereals (these are converted very quickly to glucose in the body).

- Malted products: including some cereals such as Weetabix, brown Ryvita, granary bread and malted drinks like Horlicks and Caro.

- Fermented products: including alcohol, ginger beer, vinegar and foods containing it, salad cream, baked beans, soy sauce and sourdough bread.

- Cow's milk: including most milk products including cream and most cheeses.

- Fresh fruit: including raw and stewed fruit but see below for exceptions.

- Dried fruit: very concentrated sugar.

- Nuts: especially peanuts as they contain a lot of mould.

- Smoked and cured fish and meat: including ham, bacon, smoked salmon and smoked mackerel.

- Mushrooms: avoid all fungi.

- Cola drinks: they contain caffeine as do some painkillers.

- Artificial sweeteners: these feed candida as much as sugar.

- Preservatives: yeast is involved in processing preservatives such as citric acid.

- Hot curries: these destroy good bacteria.

- Mould or damp: remove from home. (NB Plants can harbour mould.)

YOU CAN EAT:

- Yeast-free soda bread with wholemeal flour, rice cakes, oatcakes, Ryvita other than brown (but do not eat wheat if sensitive to it).

- Almond or rice milk without sugar.

- Butter in small amounts.

- Natural yogurt, cottage cheese.

- Organic lean meat, chicken, fish: all.

- All fresh vegetables: eat a large variety and good quantities too!

- Avocados.

- Lemons.

- Seeds and freshly cracked nuts.

- Fresh herbs: all.

- Eggs.

- Brown rice, millet, quinoa: eat lots for energy.

- Beans, peas, lentils.

- Tomato juice.

- Fruit teas.

- Two fruits a day: preferably less sweet ones such as grapefruit or berries but not grapes.

NB Please eat good quantities of the foods listed above to avoid fatigue.

Take supplements for a time

The diet itself will usually not be enough to kill off most of the yeast. You will need to take supplements after about a month. There are many substances that could be recommended but the most usual ones are:

- *Caprylic acid*: this is a fatty acid found in coconuts. It is less toxic than some other anti-fungals and does not kill off the good bacteria.

- Garlic: eat some raw every day.

- *Aloe vera*: this has soothing and healing properties.

- *Saccharomyces boulardii*: surprisingly this is a yeast that helps us as it is important for the formation of secretory immunoglobulin A (IgA), which is in mucous and helps ward off toxins.

- Water: drink lots while on this programme in order to flush out the candida as it dies off.

Die-off

As the candida dies off it releases toxins, which can make you feel unwell for a short time. You may have nausea, anxiety or even depression so you need to kill off the yeast slowly. Start slowly with the caprylic acid and build to a higher dose gradually. Drinking plenty of water helps flush the toxins out of your system. Taking extra vitamin C and using the herb milk thistle can help prevent this being a problem. Some nutritionists also claim that milk thistle can help protect the liver.

The good thing is that symptoms of candida can become much better after about a month and many people then feel very well. It is very important to note that this strict diet is not forever. If you do not feel any better after six weeks you should think again. This is very important.

If you do feel better but begin eating lots of sugary foods candida can regrow again quite quickly. The latest research suggests that many of these sugary foods are bad for us any-way and are implicated in type 2 diabetes, heart disease and even cancer, so it is sensible to keep away from excessive consumption. The non-sugary or starchy foods on the list, such as mushrooms, can be brought back after the yeast has been reduced.

Nutritional therapists

As there is so much to consider in relation to candida, it might be useful to work with a qualified nutritional thera-pist. If you are in the UK, look for one who is a member of the British Association for Applied Nutrition & Nutritional Therapy.

In a nutshell

- The first thing to do is to be tested for SIBO; have this treated, if necessary.

- At the same time, try giving up all wheat for a few weeks to see if you feel better.

- Test for parasites; these can exist with or without candida.

- If you suspect allergies or food intolerance, do the elimination, blood and/or pinprick tests.

- Test also for candida; if yeast overgrowth is suspected follow the anti-candida programme for a few months.

Chapter 4

REPLACING WHAT SHOULD BE IN YOUR DIGESTIVE TRACT

In order to have good digestion we need to have enough of the substances listed below. Therefore, the next step is to check for these and replace them if needed.

• Stomach acid

• Digestive enzymes

• Fibre

• The best food

Do you have enough stomach acid?

It may seem strange to be asking whether you have enough stomach acid. So often, we are told that we have too much and pharmacies are awash with pills to help us reduce it. What is going on here?

Many of us know what it feels like to have acid backing up from our stomachs. It is a horrible feeling and you just want to wash it out with water right away. When this happens, we usually assume that we have too much acid but, strangely enough, this may not be so. We *need* our stomach acid and it

63

has to be very strong. It is difficult to have too much, especially as we get older. When we get heartburn, the problem is not that we have too much acid but that we have acid *in the wrong place.*

Stomach acid should stay right there in the stomach, but when it moves up into the oesophagus, we experience this as heartburn. The acid then starts to irritate the lining of the oesophagus and cause pain and inflammation. This is because the acid has escaped from its normal home and not because we have too much of it.

Antacids everywhere

In order to stop the irritation many people buy over-the-counter antacids. These are alkalis and neutralize acid. You may know from school chemistry that if you combine an acid with an alkali you will get a salt plus water. Over-the-counter antacids are sold in high quantities and, if the problem is more serious, doctors may also give a prescription for drugs. Some of these work by stopping your body producing the acid at source. However, these medications can lead to other problems later on.

Why is low stomach acid a problem?

Although it is commonly thought that too much acid causes acid reflux and heartburn, some practitioners argue that it is caused by the valve at the top of the stomach not closing properly. Surprisingly this can be caused by having too little acid. Of course, those suffering from a hiatus hernia cannot have chronic acidity irritating the lining of their oesophagus so they may need to take antacids for a time. (Incidentally, a hiatus hernia can sometimes be helped by an adjustment from a chiropractor.) However, too many others are taking antacids for too long.

If we do not have enough stomach acid, we can't digest our food properly. This means that we can't break down protein foods like meat or fish into separate amino acids. Neither can we absorb minerals like calcium, magnesium, zinc, copper, iron and selenium properly. This can lead to all sorts of problems like osteoporosis, arthritis and even depression later on.

Another important function of stomach acid is the absorption of vitamin B12. Deficiencies of this vitamin can cause a form of anaemia, but some antacid drugs (proton pump inhibitors) can lower levels of B12 to less than 1 per cent. We also need the acid so that our stomach empties correctly.

We should care about the acid in our stomach more because it is very important to protect us from bacteria or yeasts that might arrive there. It kills them. If we don't have enough, we are less protected from conditions like gastroenteritis, *Helicobacter pylori* (*H. pylori*) infection, SIBO and parasites. Therefore, you can see that not having *enough* acid can be a problem.

Symptoms of low stomach acid

- Bloating, belching burping or wind immediately after meals.

- Feeling full after eating a few bites of food.

- Feeling that food is just sitting in the stomach and not being digested.

- Undigested food in the stool.

- Heartburn.

- Allergies.

- Vitamin B12 deficiency (vitamin B12 has many functions in the body).

- Itching of the rectum.

- Candida overgrowth.

- Iron-deficiency anaemia.

- Weak, peeling fingernails.

Acid production needs zinc

One cause of low stomach acid is a deficiency of the mineral zinc. This is quite common, especially in vegetarians as zinc is found mainly in animal foods. As non-vegetarians can also have low acid it is a good idea to be tested for this. You can ask your doctor for the test or go to a private laboratory. If low, eat more zinc-rich foods (see opposite) or take a supplement and test again a few months later.

Zinc-rich foods	
Oysters	Green peas
Ginger root	Shrimps
Lamb	Turnips
Pecan nuts	Brazil nuts
Haddock	Egg yolks

Zinc taste test

This is a simple test that gives an indication of zinc deficiency. You buy a solution, which you take according to the instructions, and then decide what the solution tastes like. Your answer will give you an indication of whether or not you are low in zinc. If you are low, you can then have a blood test done to confirm it.

Tests for stomach acid: home tests

• Dissolve a level teaspoon of bicarbonate of soda in some water and drink this on an empty stomach (so it is better to do the test first thing in the morning before you put anything into your mouth). It should make you bloat and belch within five to ten minutes. This happens because sodium bicarbonate reacts with the acid in your stomach to form carbon dioxide. You will be familiar with this gas from fizzy drinks, so you will know that it can cause belching. If you have little or no belching this indicates that you might have low stomach acid.

- Eat some beetroot and then check your urine to see if it goes a pinkish colour, which indicates low acid.

- Take some cider vinegar or lemon juice in water after food. If this eases the discomfort, you may be short of stomach acid.

The above tests give an indication of low stomach acid. They are not foolproof, but taken together they are quite useful.

Tests for stomach acid: medical tests

Other tests are available from your doctor including the Heidelberg capsule test, which must be carried out by a medical practitioner. You swallow a little radio transmitter in a small capsule about the size of a vitamin pill and this checks the stomach for acid. However, this test is not widely available in the UK.

Treatment of low stomach acid

- It is possible to buy supplements of hydrochloric acid and betaine, but discuss this with your doctor first. They should be taken just for a short time and you should not take these at all if you have acid in your oesophagus, a hiatus hernia or an ulcer.

- Taking herbal bitters is a natural way to stimulate digestion (Swedish bitters can be found in health-food stores).

- Cider vinegar in water or lemon juice in a little water can sometimes help.

- Taking vitamin C with meals can help absorption of food.

Do you have enough digestive enzymes?

Digestive enzymes are very important in helping us digest our food. These are needed to break down the food into a form that can be absorbed properly into the bloodstream. You can see the action of enzymes when you wash up greasy dishes with detergent. The enzymes in the detergent break down the large globules of fat left behind on the dish from our succulent dinner. If you look closely, you will see that when the washing up liquid is added the fat globules become much smaller. The enzymes in our mouth and enzymes in other parts of our body work in a similar way, breaking down the food for digestion. For example, the saliva in our mouth contains the enzyme amylase, which is needed to break down sugars and starches.

Enzymes are also produced lower down our digestive tract. Our pancreas squirts out pancreatic enzymes on to the food to break it down.

The suffix 'ase' shows us that a substance is an enzyme: amylase found in our saliva and in the small intestine digests carbohydrate; protease helps us digest protein; lipase helps us digest fats; and lactase helps us digest lactose, the sugar in milk.

The enzymes produced by our pancreas are very important in other ways too because, amazingly, they also seek out and destroy cancer cells. They do this by dissolving the coating that cancer cells use to protect themselves. So you can see how important these are to our health in general.

Most raw foods contain digestive enzymes, which are destroyed when cooking, so it is a good idea to include some raw foods in your diet every day. However, until you are better do not eat very hard and fibrous raw foods such as carrots. You might like to try lightly blending whole vegetables to a liquid. As this still includes fibre it is not the same as juicing.

Symptoms of low levels of digestive enzymes

- Undigested food in the stools.
- Bloating within three hours after eating.
- Loose stools.
- Stools containing mucous.
- Abdominal cramping.
- Pale tan-coloured stools (not digesting fat).
- Acid reflux/heartburn.
- Stools that float because you are lacking in the enzymes that digest fat (lipase).

When we are under stress we do not produce as many enzymes as we need and this makes us less able to digest our food properly.

Tests for low pancreatic enzymes

A stool test can be carried via a nutritional therapist. Choose one who is a member of the British Association for Applied Nutrition and Nutritional Therapy.

How to improve your levels of digestive enzymes

- Don't drink with meals.

- Eat better quality foods as outlined in this book (see Chapter 7).

- Take supplements of digestive enzymes for a time (vegetarian options are available in health-food shops).

- Get tested for zinc deficiency, as zinc is needed to make enzymes; if low, take supplements and retest.

- Add to your diet supplements of enzymes such as bromelain, papaya or pancreatic enzymes (which can be bought from health-food shops).

Although you can supplement enzymes for a time, some practitioners argue that we can become too used to these and then need to supplement more and more. However, they can be useful in the short term until our natural digestive function improves. They can be bought in health-food shops and different types are available. Look for those that contain amylase, protease and lipase; these enzymes break down carbohydrate, protein and fat in that order.

Do you eat enough fibre

Could you be eating too little fibre? It used to be thought that the fibrous parts of foods were not important because they did not seem to be digested but we now know that fibre is essential for good digestion. Fibre works in a very interesting way: it attracts water like blotting paper, and so helps bulk up and soften the stool, making it easier to pass. You might think that it's odd that it can help both consti-pation and diarrhoea but it can. This is because it soaks up the excess fluid making loose stools more solid while adding fluid to hard stools. Fibre is a prime supporter for our health as it has many functions: it combines with toxins and takes them out of the body; it helps us excrete excess cholesterol and excess oestrogen; and it helps feed beneficial bacteria.

Many foods contain no fibre

You can see, therefore, that fibre is very important. The problem is that many foods contain almost no fibre. This applies to some good foods that are highly nutritious in other ways like meat, chicken, fish and eggs. Of course, we do need these but if we don't balance them with foods that are more fibrous we can end up with constipation. Non-nutritious foods that lack fibre are those made from white flour like bread, pasta, cakes, biscuits, pastries and sweets. You can see therefore that it is very easy to have a very low-fibre diet if you do not think about what you are eating. Low-fibre diets are often the norm as people become more reliant on wheat-based foods like pasta and bread, and eat fewer fruits and vegetables.

Constipation is not the only problem caused by not eating enough fibre. It doesn't end there. Straining in the toilet itself can lead to other conditions such as haemorrhoids (piles), varicose veins or even diverticulitis, where the colon bulges out into pockets. Food can be trapped in these, causing pain and inflammation. You can see why it is important to keep your motions soft.

Types of fibre

There are two types of fibre: soluble and insoluble. Soluble fibre dissolves in water and acts like a gel in the body, and so it is very soothing for the digestive system. For example, if you put some flaxseeds in a glass of water and leave them, the mixture will look like a jelly when you return. This jelly-like substance helps the passage of wastes in the digestive tract as it attracts water, and plumps up and softens the stool.

Foods high in soluble fibre include:

- Brussels sprouts;
- other green vegetables;
- root vegetables such as turnips, carrots and sweet potatoes;

- white potatoes;
- fruits such as bananas and apples;
- linseed (flaxseed);
- porridge;
- cucumber;
- pear;
- psyllium, which can be bought in health-food shops (add lots of water).

Many vegetables combine high soluble fibre with lots of water so these are very helpful. Cabbage, broccoli and cucumber come into this category. These also have important anti-cancer properties so making them a big part of your diet will help in more ways than one. If you have had problem digesting foods like cabbage and broccoli in the past, the overall programme outlined in this book should help.

The diet described here should help with many problems as it includes vegetables as a staple along with some fruit. Making soup with vegetables is also good because you are combining fibre with lots of water.

Don't use bran

It has often been thought that adding lots of wheat bran to your diet can help constipation. This is not a good idea because wheat bran is harsher on the system. It can also bind to much-needed minerals and take them out of the body (so children should not be given cereals with added bran). If you have wheat intolerance, bran of this kind will make the problem worse. It is also not a good idea to eat lots of wholemeal bread for fibre.

Try not to increase your fibre all at once: start with a low amount and increase it slowly. Make sure you have enough water in your diet to soften the fibre, otherwise you could get a mass of hard matter in the gut. Eat healthy fats and oils to help keep the digestive tract well lubricated (see Chapter 7).

In a nutshell

- For good digestion, we need to have adequate levels of important substances.

- We need to have enough stomach acid; without it, we cannot break down protein foods or absorb minerals.

- We also need to have enough digestive enzymes; if necessary, these can be supplemented for a time.

- Fibre is also needed, especially the soluble type from vegetables and fruit.

- In addition to this, we need to eat the natural, unprocessed diet that has sustained us for thousands of years.

- Ideally we should cook fresh food from scratch.

Chapter 5

RE-INOCULATING YOURSELF WITH GOOD BACTERIA

Bacteria may not be the first thing that you think about when looking at digestive health, but we have a huge amount of these in our gut. Research has shown that they do a wonderful job in keeping us healthy. In fact, our digestive system contains more bacteria than cells in our body, and we have around 500 different strains living in our digestive tract.

Added together, there are over 100 trillion bacteria weighing about four pounds making their home there. Some of these bacteria are harmful but others are very protective and are good for us in many ways. These are often called 'beneficial' or 'friendly' bacteria or 'good gut flora'.

The importance of good bacteria in helping with the symptoms of IBS

Good bacteria or probiotics can help the symptoms of IBS according to a study published in the *World Journal of Gastroenterology*.[11] This was a review of fifteen randomized, placebo-controlled trials that studied 1,793 patients. The researchers looked at distension, bloating and flatulence, comparing those given probiotics to those given a placebo (a dummy pill). They found that those taking the probiotics had less pain and the other symptoms were less severe. This was a good piece of research for two reasons: firstly, it was a review providing information from many studies; and secondly, the researchers used randomized controlled trials, which are seen as the gold standard of research methods.

Have you lost your good bacteria?

When we are born, our digestive tract is sterile and, if we are breastfed, the good bacteria are introduced into our systems from the milk. Of course, many of us were not breastfed so would not have had this advantage and probably had quite a few courses of antibiotics as children. These drugs have undoubtedly saved many lives but the current thinking is that they have been used too much. This is because they kill off good bacteria as well as the ones that cause the problems. It was for this reason that in previous years doctors used to give probiotics alongside antibiotics to make up for the good bacteria that were killed off.

Another source of antibiotics is those given to cows and chickens, sometimes routinely, to prevent infection. These can also kill off beneficial bacteria and indeed some doctors have become concerned about this. Other dangers to our good bacteria are chlorine in tap water, smoking, stress and, strangely enough, flying too much.

An interesting fact about these bacteria is that different strains have different functions in the body. You can see, therefore, how important it is to try to keep these in good shape and replace those lost by the use of antibiotics or other factors. Beneficial bacteria do not just help prevent IBS: they affect our health in all sorts of other ways.

Bacterial benefits

- They prevent yeasts and bad bacteria taking hold.

- They stop our gut lining being damaged. This is very important because if this occurs, substances can leak into the bloodstream that should not be there. When this happens, the body can set up an immune response and this can lead to autoimmune conditions like rheumatoid arthritis, thyroiditis and scleroderma.

- They act like our own vitamin factory producing the vitamins B1, B2, B3, folic acid and vitamin B12, and help the production of other nutrients such as vitamin D and vitamin K, which is important for good bone density.

- They regulate cholesterol and triglycerides, and help the immune system.

- Some of them make minerals like calcium, copper, iron, magnesium and manganese more available to the body.

- They help to protect us from food poisoning.

- They help us to digest our food.

- They stop bad bacteria and yeasts gaining hold as they produce antibiotic and anti-fungal substances.

- They help us to digest lactose, the sugar in milk. This means that people with lactose intolerance can often still eat yogurt and other cultured milks.

- They protect our immune system. In fact, we know that 85 per cent of our immune system is located in our digestive tract.

Re-inoculating yourself with good bacteria

Adding back: supplements

Beneficial bacteria can be bought in powder or capsule form and taken as supplements, in which case they are called 'probiotics'. There are a great many on the market so you need to buy them from a reputable company.

It is a good idea to aim to replenish our good bacteria quickly, and the simplest way to begin is by taking supplements. You might think that it is better to use probiotic foods such as kefir. I agree that it is usually better to get what we need from food rather than pills but, in this case, we need to replenish the gut flora quickly. Depending on food alone might take too long. Also, shop-bought yogurts do not always contain the amount of bacteria that they should. It is best, therefore, to use supplements for a while and then keep the bacteria topped up by eating lots of probiotic-rich foods. After a few weeks on supplements, you can use fermented foods to keep the probiotics going.

The supplement should contain billions of bacteria, especially *Lactobacillus acidophilus* and *Bifidobacterium*. Another useful bacterium is *Saccharomyces boulardii*. This is yeast but a good one this time as it helps us produce secretory IgA. This is part of our gut mucous, and protects us from bacteria and yeasts. You can test for this by collecting your saliva at home and sending it to a laboratory via a nutritionist. One study published in the *Journal of Clinical Gastroenterology* found that this improved the quality of life for IBS sufferers better than a placebo.[12]

Adding back: foods

Quite a few foods contain good bacteria naturally. These foods have been fermented and are often very pleasant to take. Many societies ferment foods in order to preserve them and some of them can last for many months. For example, in very cold climates such as parts of Russia it is not possible to grow vegetables in winter so people ferment foods like cabbage in order to have them throughout the year. Fermenting traditions vary: in the Middle East, they ferment kefir, in Austria they have yogurt; India has lassi; and Israel has leben. Originally, they may not have known how beneficial they are but these foods contain large amounts of good bacteria and so are of great benefit to our digestive systems.

Be careful not to confuse fermented foods with pickled foods. Pickled foods like pickled cucumber and onions use vinegar rather than probiotic cultures and are not as beneficial as fermented foods.

Foods that contain good bacteria

You can use probiotic supplements for a few months and then eat foods that contain good bacteria after that. Below are some suggestions.

Yogurt

This is the fermented food that is most familiar to us. In the West, sales of yogurt have increased massively over the last few decades but it was always popular in other countries. It can be made with different milks that are produced from cows, sheep, goats, soya, rice, nuts and coconut. Many of the more unusual varieties are available from health-food shops. It is not a good idea to eat highly sweetened or artificially flavoured or coloured yogurts. Plain ones are better, and buy organic if you can. Fortunately, yogurt is also easy to make at home and yogurt enthusiasts usually say that this tastes much better than that bought in shops. If you do this, you can choose whatever milk you like, including almond or coconut. Try not to use milks with added sugar, such as some types of rice milk and soya milk.

There is an argument that humans should not drink milk at all. In fact, we are the only species that drinks the milk of another animal and, in many parts of the world, no milk is drunk after weaning. Some practitioners recommend cutting out all milk but others feel that sheep's or goat's milk is not as bad as cow's milk.

Kefir

This runny fermented food comes from the Caucasus Mountains in Russia. The word '*kefir*' is Turkish and means 'good feeling'. It is made from special grains, which can be bought online. It can be grown on ordinary milk or, for those who are dairy sensitive, the good news is that you can grow it on rice milk, coconut milk or soya milk.

One study published in the *Journal of the American Dietetic Association* found that kefir improved the digestion of lactose, which is the sugar in milk. In addition, it reduced flatulence by 54 per cent to 84 per cent relative to milk.[13]

Kefir is very easy to make. All you need to do is put the grains into a quart of milk, which could be dairy, soya or coconut, and leave it in a warm place for a few days. It should begin to look like a junket and taste tangy. Then you strain it and add fresh milk. This needs to be carried out two or three times until it thickens. After that, it can be kept in the fridge. When you buy the grains instructions are included. Don't expect it to become solid like commercial yogurt as it tends to be much looser and more liquid. It's extremely pleasant tangy taste is very refreshing, especially on hot days.

Fermented cabbage

This has been eaten in Russia for hundreds of years. The process of fermenting vegetables has allowed people living in cold climates to be able to eat them throughout the whole year. '*Sauerkraut*' is a German word that just means sour cabbage. We now know that it contains high levels of good bacteria. It is not difficult to make and can be a delicious accompaniment to a meal. All you do is chop the cabbage into small pieces or strips, add in salt, put it in a bowl or crock and then squeeze it with your hands until some juice comes out. Cover with a plate, leaving a small space for gas to escape, and leave for several days or a couple of weeks, making sure the cabbage is submerged in its own juices.

Do not eat more than a few teaspoons of sauerkraut at a time to begin with as the beneficial bacteria can be quite potent.

Prebiotic foods

Prebiotics are foods that feed the probiotics or beneficial bacteria such as *Lactobacillus acidophilus* and *Bifidobacterium* in the colon or large bowel. We have seen how important probiotics are for good digestion, and in order to grow and flourish these bacteria need food just like other living things. Probiotics need to be taken regularly in order for them to stay around but prebiotics do not have this disadvantage. As well as encouraging the good bacteria to grow, they are more stable.

The main prebiotics are non-digestible sugars called 'oligo-saccharides'. The food that contains the highest amount of prebiotics is raw chicory but this is not something we eat often. Fortunately, some more common foods also contain it. These are Jerusalem artichoke, raw garlic, raw onion, cooked onion, raw asparagus, green tea, leeks, kefir and bananas. Other sources are fructooligosaccharides (FOS) and inulin, which can be taken as supplements. A few studies have suggested that low doses of prebiotics may improve symptoms of IBS.

If you find that you get wind and bloating when you begin taking prebiotics, start slowly and work up to a higher dose. These problems usually go after about a week.

In a nutshell

- Beneficial bacteria are very important for digestion.

- Research has shown that they can help the symptoms of IBS.

- Antibiotics can kill off many of these while we are being treated for bacterial infections.

- We can replace these with capsules to begin with. These should contain billions of bacteria.

- After that we should eat foods that are high in these bacteria such as kefir and sauerkraut.

- Kefir and yogurt can be made from non-dairy milks such as coconut.

- Try also to eat foods that feed these good bacteria.

Chapter 6

REPAIRING YOUR DIGESTIVE TRACT

After working through Chapters 3 to 5, your digestive tract may be slightly inflamed or damaged. This can be helped by eating anti-inflammatory foods like oily fish and turmeric. However, if candida or parasites have damaged the gut lining it can become more permeable. This is often called 'leaky gut'.

What is a leaky gut?

I know that leaky gut is an odd-sounding phrase and might make you imagine a digestive system that is full of holes. Although it is not as dramatic as it sounds, it is actually a little like this. Another name for leaky is *intestinal gut permeability*. What this means is that the cells that line the small intestine allow things to pass through because they are wider apart than they should be.

The cells in the walls of that part of the body should be very close together, very tight. That is why the connection between the cells is called a 'tight junction'. This tightness is needed to stop certain substances from getting into the bloodstream. The problem is that this tight junction can become damaged: it becomes irritated and inflamed, and the junctions loosen up, making it more permeable.

All sorts of things can make this happen, including chemicals from the environment, junk foods, yeasts, parasites and wheat-based foods. Therefore, this normally tight junction becomes permeable and is no longer the powerful gatekeeper that it should be. This allows undigested food particles, bacteria and fungi to gain access to the bloodstream and do damage. If you have a leaky gut, you may not feel anything very much and there will not be much to see if you have a colonoscopy. However, it can still cause many problems including some that would seem unrelated, such as autoimmune conditions where the body attacks itself.

IBS and leaky gut

Leaky gut and IBS are associated. One study found that 39 per cent of the sample of IBS patients had this problem, particularly the ones whose main symptom was diarrhoea. In fact one American doctor, Dr Sherry Rogers, has stated that 'most IBS is leaky gut in disguise and is totally curable'.[14]

One study in the *American Journal of Gastroenterology* found that permeability of the colon was significantly increased in those with IBS-D, the diarrhoea type of IBS, compared to a control group who did not suffer from these conditions.[15]

What causes leaky gut?

There are various ways that the gut can become more permeable. These are:

- *Yeast overgrowth* (see the candida section of Chapter 3): as always, we need to look for this and treat it as it can break down the brush borders (the villi or small hairs in the digestive tract).

- *Parasites*: *Blastocystis hominis*, amoebas, salmonella, *Shigella*, *Giardia*, and *Helicobacter pylori* can irritate the gut lining and cause problems.

- *Chronic stress*: see Chapter 10 for ideas on how to deal with this.

- *Alcohol*: this can cause leaky gut as it lowers our production of anti-inflammatory chemicals called prostaglandins.

- *Medical drugs*: including non-steroidal anti-inflammatories such as aspirin.

- *Poor food choices*: processed foods in particular should be avoided, as well as other foods such as wheat and dairy that the individual cannot tolerate well.

What happens next?

When our gut becomes permeable or leaky, things that should not get into the bloodstream gain admittance. Our immune system then senses that there are foreign invaders lurking about and sets up an immune attack. This then activates antibodies and white blood cells, and the site becomes inflamed.

In addition to this, many naturopathic practitioners and some doctors think that a leaky gut can give rise to other conditions. These are called autoimmune diseases, where the body starts to attack itself. You will probably have heard of some of these such as thyroiditis, multiple sclerosis, where the myelin sheath around the nerves is attacked, fibromyalgia, rheumatoid arthritis, where the joints are attacked, Graves' disease of the thyroid, scleroderma and many more. These are not digestive problems as such but arise from damage to the digestive system. This means that repairing your digestive tract can go a long way to preventing you becoming ill in many other parts of your body. Some practitioners would even say that our health in general begins in the gut.

Symptoms of a leaky gut

The digestive symptoms of a leaky gut are very similar to the symptoms of other conditions:

- Wind or flatulence
- Bloating
- Abdominal cramps
- Fatigue
- Rashes
- Joint pains

The thinking is that leaky gut is the cause of food allergies because when these substances get into the bloodstream the immune system starts to attack them. However, it does not stop there. The foreign invaders can use the bloodstream to travel all over and attach to other parts of the body. For example, they could attach to a knee joint causing inflammation. One nutritionist has argued that every time you eat a particular food you will have inflammation in the joints within forty-eight hours.[16] The good news, however, is that these conditions can be helped by healing the gut.

Strangely enough, while you might think that if the gut is leaky it can absorb more nutrients, this is the opposite of what happens. A leaky gut stops us absorbing some nutrients because the carrier proteins needed to transport them into the blood are also damaged. This can lead to vitamin and mineral deficiencies even if you eat a good diet.

Testing for a leaky gut

This is a simple urine test where you collect a sample at home and send it to a laboratory for analysis. This can be carried out via a qualified nutritionist. You are asked to drink two solutions, lactulose and mannitol, and a urine sample is taken after six hours. If you are fine, the mannitol should be found in the urine but not the lactulose. Your gut should not absorb the lactulose easily. If it does, this is a sign that your gut is leaky.

On the other hand, the mannitol *should* be absorbed easily. If it is not then this shows that the right nutrients are not getting through to your bloodstream. If neither gets through you should be tested for coeliac disease. As the test uses sorbitol, xylitol and lactulose, you should not take it if you are intolerant to these substances.

If you do have leaky-gut syndrome you need to find out why. Therefore, the next step is to look at the stool to find out what is lurking in there. As mentioned, substances that can cause leaky gut are yeasts, parasites and unhealthy bacteria.

The stool test also looks for good amounts of substances that you do need, such as digestive enzymes. One such test is the CDSA (comprehensive digestive stool analysis) but by now you may have dealt with the possible causes like candida.

The programme outlined in this book should deal with the causes of a leaky gut. After dealing with possible candida, parasites, etc., you then take steps to deal with any inflammation or leaky gut.

How to heal a leaky gut

The good news is that there are many foods that can help reduce inflammation and heal the digestive tract. You can use supplements for a few weeks or months and then the best foods should be eaten to keep the system healthy. Below is a list of the important ones:

- *Essential fatty acids*: these are omega-3 from fish oil and omega-6 from nuts and seeds. When eating nuts and seeds it is very important to grind them very finely, as they can be difficult to digest. Of course, we also need to cut out all processed fats and oils such as sunflower, canola (another name for rapeseed) and margarine, and all foods made from these (see Chapter 7).

- *Natural coconut oil*: although not an essential oil, natural coconut fat is good for digestion.

- *Zinc-rich foods*: zinc is high in seafood, beef and lamb, sesame seeds, lentils and turkey. As zinc deficiency is common, it is a good idea to be tested for this. Zinc is very important for good digestion because it is needed to make stomach acid and helps repair the gut lining. If you need a supplement, zinc carnosine is good for healing the gut. Nutritionist Sherry Rogers recommends 75 mg twice daily.[17]

- *Turmeric*: one of the most potent natural anti-inflammatories in existence is curcumin from turmeric. Be careful not to confuse this with cumin as this is a different plant. One study found that turmeric was as effective as cortisone itself. It works by making our bodies produce more cortisone naturally and makes the body more sensitive to it.

- As well as reducing inflammation, turmeric can also help with the symptoms of IBS. One trial of 207 volunteers carried out over eight weeks gave groups one or two tablets of turmeric extract. The results showed that IBS decreased significantly in both groups by 41 per cent and 57 per cent.[18] Turmeric powder can be added to soups, stews and other dishes, and has a very mild curry flavour. As it can be difficult to absorb it is important to eat it with pepper and some fat. Organic turmeric powder is best and can be bought from supermarkets or you can buy it fresh. Have it most days.

- *Gamma oryzanol*: this comes from rice bran oil and is useful for helping IBS and other conditions. Take 100 mg three times a day for at least three weeks.

Healing herbs

- *Deglycyrrhizinated liquorice (DGL)*: this has been used for digestive health for a long time and helps form a protective barrier against inflammation.

- *Aloe vera*: this is a soothing herb.

- *Marshmallow*: This is not the white fluffy sweet but the herb, which helps soothe inflamed tissue.

In a nutshell

- Now you need to deal with any inflammation or possible leaky gut.

- You can do a test for leaky gut or you can just take steps to heal it anyway.

- After dealing with the conditions in Chapters 3 to 5 you can use foods and supplements to repair it.

- Eating the best diet as suggested in Chapter 7 should help to keep your digestive tract healthy.

Chapter 7

EATING THE BEST FOOD FOR DIGESTIVE HEALTH

Do you ever feel that you are being given lots of conflicting advice about what to eat and what not to eat? Do you feel that you are being bombarded with masses of different information about food from different sources and don't know what to believe? I know that many do. From being told to eat low-fat then high-fat foods, margarine then butter, vegetarian or not, high carbohydrate then low carbohydrate, everyone seems to be giving advice. No wonder there is such confusion. What is the truth and how do we know what to believe?

This chapter will tell you the truth. It describes the best way of eating to keep us healthy and free from digestive problems and all sorts of diseases. When I give this information to clients, they say it makes sense to them. The food choices become obvious because we ate this way since time began. The good news is that the best diet should protect you from all sorts of conditions, not just IBS. You may think that this is too good to be true but most diseases are actually caused by poor food. We are not talking here about fault: we are talking about cause. Very many people really want to eat well but they are led astray by marketing, advertising and false claims.

What is wrong with our diet?

Many of us are undernourished

That statement may surprise you. When I give talks, I always ask the audience if anyone thinks they are undernourished and they all laugh, especially the women. This is because many of us think that we are too heavy and therefore well nourished. Unfortunately, this is not so. It is possible to be overfed and undernourished at the same time, and many people in Western societies have this problem. Much of the food we are eating is high in calories but low in vitamins, minerals, essential fats and the other chemicals in plants that prevent disease. These are called phytonutrients or plant nutrients and there are thousands. Every part of our body, including our bones, blood, hormones, hair, brain and even our genes, is made from nutrients. We cannot be really well if we are undernourished.

New foods on the block

We are undernourished because much of our food is lacking in nutrients. This is very different from the food of yesteryear, which is one reason why we find it so difficult to digest. What we are now eating is vastly different from what we ate for most of our history and what we consumed as we developed as a species. Our ancestors would not recognize many of the foods we find in the modern supermarket; foods that have been so stripped of nutrition that often we can't use them to build health.

You might think that no one in the West is undernourished. We don't appear to be because our supermarkets are full of every tasty morsel you can imagine. The problem is that so much of that is not giving us much at all except calories. It is heavily processed and does not contain the nutrients that it should.

Good digestion depends on nourishing food. One study published in the *Journal of Gastrointestinal Liver Diseases* (Chirila *et al.*, 2012) found that in their sample those with IBS were more likely to eat canned food, processed meat, pulses, whole cereals, confectionary, fruit compotes and herbal teas. It is not clear which of these might be the greatest cause of IBS but the research does suggest that eating cereals and processed or canned foods is not doing the best for our digestion.

We have been on this planet for thousands of years but many of the foods we are eating today were introduced only in the last hundred. We evolved eating fresh, natural, unprocessed foods. Now we eat highly processed new foods and this leads to poor health and poor digestion.

Many of us do try to eat a good healthy diet but so much of the foods that are sold as 'healthy' are in fact quite the opposite. You might think that it would be illegal to sell unhealthy food but this is not the case. As far as the law is concerned, food has to be safe but not necessarily healthy.

This means that it cannot contain dirt, poisons or bacteria but it doesn't have to be good for us and much of it isn't.

Food processing affects digestion

You might argue that people all over the world have developed on different foods. Eskimos ate whale blubber, Hindus are vegetarian, those living by the sea ate mainly fish, and the fact is that people ate what was there, what was available to them. Does this mean then that we can just eat anything or that we can adapt to any type of food? I am sure you know that the answer is 'no'. Although these people ate different foods, they were all natural, whole and not processed. The big difference between what we eat now, particularly in the West, and what we ate traditionally is the processing.

We have changed ordinary food so much that it is as nothing found in nature. This is true of processed vegetable oils like sunflower and corn, white breads and pastas, refined sugar, boxed cereals and so on. The way we are producing food nowadays is not the way it was produced in former times. Actually, in the past it wasn't *produced* at all. It was just there. We simply ate what we could hunt or get from foraging. Strangely enough, we therefore often had a much more varied diet than we do today.

The words 'balanced diet' tell us nothing

We are often told to 'eat a balanced diet'. However, what does this really mean? Actually, it means very little. The phrase is true by definition and means almost nothing. It does not tell us what constitutes a balanced diet. Many think of a balanced diet as a bit of everything in the supermarket. This could not be further from the truth. In addition, what seems to be a balanced diet to one person might be a very poor diet to another. How much sugar, if any, should you eat on a balanced diet and how much meat? Can you have crisps on a balanced diet? If so, how many packets?

What is 'moderation'?

Another thing that you hear people say is that we should eat 'everything in moderation'. This again does not tell us very much. Some diabetic people are told to eat refined sugar 'in moderation'. What does this mean? To me it means practically none; to others it might mean quite a lot.

You might also hear some food professionals say that there are 'no bad foods, just bad diets'. What they mean by this is that you can eat everything as long as there is not too much of the less valuable foods. I do not agree with this. In my opinion, there *are* bad foods. These are the highly processed foods that are made in factories. They may be quite tasty but they are very different from what we ate traditionally. An example of this is processed oils, which are discussed fully overleaf: we should not have any of those. The diet that our ancestors ate since time began is the right diet for us today.

Why is food not as it should be?

- *Food processing*: we have taken many natural, ordinary foods and changed them into something never seen before. This applies to oils, wheat and the farming of fish. For example, when fish are farmed, they may not be given the right diet. Instead of the plankton or little fish that they need, they might be fed a diet based on cereals. This then changes the type of fat the fish contains. It will have less omega-3 and so be less nutritious for us.

- *Food storage*: food is often stored for long periods and travels long distances before we get it. When this happens, it deteriorates and loses nutrients.

- *Farming practices*: modern farming practices frequently leave much to be desired. Often the soil in which the food is grown has not been re-mineralized. As plants use up the nutrients in the soil these need to be replenished. In the past farmers would rotate the crops so that one year they might sow potatoes and another year a different vegetable because different vegetables take different nutrients from the soil. This happens much less so nowadays. Much of our food does not contain the minerals that it should. If we look at zinc, for example, we see that this is needed, along with vitamin B6 to produce the stomach acid necessary for digestion. However, many of us are low in this. Research has shown that zinc deficiency is the most common micronutrient deficiency in world crops, with approximately one-third of the world's population zinc deficient.[20] Organically grown food is better as it tends to be higher in nutrients and, of course, it does not have pesticide residues.

- *Food choices and marketing*: many people just like unhealthy foods and marketing encourages this. It is the unhealthy foods that tend to be advertised, rather than the natural healthy foods like fresh fruit and vegetables. Many of these heavily promoted foods do nothing but provide empty (but tasty) calories.

What about milk?

Do you like a cappuccino? I certainly do, even though they are made with milk so I often wonder if I should be drinking them. There is so much debate about whether milk is good for us or not. Milk has traditionally been seen as healthy, with advertisers using the slogan, 'Drinka Pinta Milka Day'. However, many nutritionists and nutritional doctors are advising that milk is not a good food for the following reasons:

- It contains the protein casein. This can be difficult to digest for some people.

- Many people do not have enough of the enzyme lactase to digest lactose, which is the sugar in milk.

- Milk is apparently full of growth hormones. Some claim that this is associated with the high incidence of breast cancer that we are now seeing.

The best way to find out how milk affects you is to cut it out for a few weeks and see how you feel. If you feel different, reintroduce it again and see if your symptoms return. If they do, cut it out. If you are worried about not getting enough calcium, you can be reassured that there is enough of this in other foods.

Excess salt

The modern diet is loaded with salt. It is added to most processed foods such as crisps, savoury snacks and just about every food that you do not make yourself. This is very different to how we ate for thousands of years. If we go back as far as the Stone Age and even later, where would we have found the salt? There is some naturally in fish and a few vegetables but we had a fraction of the amount we have today.

One of the problems with this is not just that we eat too much salt or sodium but that we eat too little potassium. Sodium and potassium have to be in balance. In the Stone Age, we ate five to ten times more potassium than sodium but now the average American diet contains just half as much potassium as sodium. Foods high in potassium are mainly fresh fruits and vegetables (without added salt) and, in former times, these would have made up the largest part of our diet. These should still make up the bulk of our diet today. Unfortunately, this is not the case.

Add in more potassium

So, in order to get the balance right, cut down your intake of salty foods and add lots of vegetables and some fruit. Vegetables are actually more important than fruit as some fruits are high in natural sugars. Berries are the best fruit as these contain the most antioxidants. It is best to eat fruit away from meals as when it is eaten with other food it can sit in the intestines and ferment, possibly causing wind and bloating.

Remember that there can be a lot of salt in foods that don't taste particularly salty such as bread, so it is best to read labels. If you are tempted by very salty foods you can help redress the balance by eating more fruit and vegetables at your next meal, gaining extra potassium, while cutting right back on the salt.

Sugar, sugar everywhere

How much refined sugar do you think we should be eating a day? One teaspoon? Six teaspoons? I would say none. This might surprise you because we are so used to eating sugar in one form or another. By sugar, I mean the white crystalline substance that we consume in desserts, sweets, cakes and biscuits, and which we put in our tea and coffee, and not the natural sugars in vegetables. The chemical name is sucrose and we should try not to eat this at all. Sucrose does nothing for our health, and one nutritionist has said that it is the biggest cause of health problems today. This might surprise you because we are now so used to having it.

The truth is that this form of sugar is completely new to our diet as it is only recently that we have been able to isolate it from sugar beet and sugar cane. Before that the only sweetener we had was honey and that was quite difficult to gather.

Have we been too clever?

It seems that we have. We have been too clever in taking out the white crystalline stuff from sugar beet and sugar cane, which concentrates the sugar. We would never be able to eat this amount of sugar in its natural form. The problem is that it is added to just about everything that we find in the shops. You know of course that it is in cakes, biscuits, desserts and sweets, but it can also be found in just about every factory-made food. This ranges from soups to ready meals to chopped herring, meat dishes and even bread. Apparently, there is more sugar in tomato ketchup than ice cream!

Most people are aware that eating too much sugar can lead to type 2 diabetes, the incidence of which has sky-rocketed, but this is not all. Sugar is implicated in the sharp rise in many other conditions such as heart disease and cancer, but this book is about digestion so we will look at how this is affected by this white crystalline sweetener.

It may be difficult to cut out sugar but I urge you to try. The rewards can be fantastic. It is good to know that you can lose a sweet tooth: after not eating sugar for a while, you begin to lose your taste for it and foods that you craved before no longer appeal. In fact you may now find them sickly and oversweet.

How sugar affects digestion

- Sugar feeds yeasts and causes an overgrowth of candida.

- It uses up our stores of important nutrients. We need B vitamins and minerals to metabolize sugar but it does not contain any nutrients itself. One of these minerals is zinc and this is needed to make stomach acid, along with vitamin B6.

- It makes us less hungry for foods that are more nutritious.

- It can cause low blood sugar a few hours after eating, which makes us want to eat more high sugar foods again a few hours later.

What should we be eating?

When I give talks to the public, I ask the audience to imagine that they have become stranded on a deserted island. I then ask them to think about what they would eat if that happened.

Some say 'coconuts', but I hope the island they have landed on is a little more fertile than that. Others say fruit, vegetables, nuts, fish, animals or eggs, in short whatever is available.

Although thankfully we are not in that situation now, we should be following this type of diet all the time. It is a diet of natural, whole, unprocessed foods, eaten fresh and as nature intended.

The natural food we ate until a few hundred years ago

sustained us and, despite all the hardships in the earliest times, we survived as a species. But don't worry, I am not saying that we should go hunting or foraging for berries: I am saying that the type of food we eat should be as similar to natural food as we can make it. Our genes have not changed in that time and we have not adapted to the new foods. Ideally, our food should be natural, organic and whole. For example, a whole apple is better than apple pie or even apple juice, our fish should be fresh and natural rather than smoked or tinned, and our fruit and vegetables should not be full of pesticides.

Although we have discussed in Chapters 3 to 6 what we need to do for specific problems, good digestion depends on what we eat overall. The aim of this chapter is to show you what the right diet contains and why. Our digestive system does not stand alone: it is part of our whole body and to strengthen it we need to make our whole system healthier and function better overall. The rewards gained from doing this can be amazing. Food is the key to the health of every part of our body. If you eat the right foods, you will be giving every part of your body the best chance of being healthy. Genes play a part but we now know that the right foods can affect how these genes are expressed.

Looking at the best diet for us

The best diet for us is the one that we ate before the advent of food processing. This means fresh organic vegetables, some fruit, organic meat and chicken, fish, eggs, nuts and seeds, and perhaps healthy grains like lentils and quinoa. The food should be fresh and not fried, smoked or have added chemicals. If you are not sure if a particular food is nutritious, ask yourself what has been done to it. A fresh carrot will just have been pulled from the soil whereas a packet of white pasta has all the nutrients taken out when the germ and bran was stripped from the starch. It has then undergone many processes to make it look the way it does. You can see then that it ends up as a very different food than it was originally.

Vegetables are by far the most important and valuable of all foods. They should be eaten at every meal. One reason is that they contain many vitamins and minerals but the latest research has shown that they also contain other substances that have a profound effect on our health. These are phyto-chemicals, from the Greek word '*phyto*' meaning 'plant', and vegetables contain many thousands of these. We now know that these have amazing anti-cancer properties and can protect us against many different types of other illnesses such as heart disease, eye diseases and a whole host of other illnesses.

Eat a rainbow

In particular, the pigments in coloured fruits and vegetables contain thousands of antioxidant compounds that can help deal with what are called free radicals. These are unbalanced atoms that lack an electron and so try to 'steal' one from another atom. The other atom in turn tries to 'steal' another and then chaos results. Antioxidants in foods donate the electrons, increasing the atoms' stability. Vegetables are full of these and other anti-cancer factors so they should make up the bulk of our diet.

Five-a-day is not enough

Some people think that they eat 'lots of vegetables' but what they really mean is that they eat something like peas and carrots with their evening meal. This is not enough. In fact, five-a-day is not enough. We need to eat many more than that to be as healthy as possible. Vegetables contain lots of 'phytonutrients' plant chemicals like beta-carotene, lutein, zeaxanthin in yellow pigments, flavonoids and so on. Literally thousands of these plant chemicals are beneficial so vegetables need to figure highly in our diets.

A great way to use vegetables is to make soup. You might think that it is a nuisance to make carrots in one pot and broccoli in another pot. And it is! However, if you put them all into a soup you get the benefit of them all together. Another good reason to have soup is that when foods are eaten together you have the benefit of synergy. This means that when you combine two fruits or vegetables the power of the combination is greater than the sum of the two alone.

Fruit

Fruit is very nutritious and the colour pigments contain important antioxidants, which can help prevent all sorts of diseases like cancer and heart disease, and eye problems like cataracts. They even help slow down the ageing process! However, for some people fruit can be difficult to digest when eaten with other foods or with meals because it ferments easily and can cause wind and bloating. So try eating fruit on its own until your digestive system is working more efficiently. This could be as a snack between meals but do not eat too much at once, though, as this can raise blood sugar too high too quickly. Fruit is good but only eat a few pieces per day.

Which protein should we choose?

As well as fruits and vegetables, we need good sources of protein, which is needed for growth and repair, including to the digestive tract. It also has many other functions in the body. The best sources are uncontaminated, organic meat, fish and eggs for non-vegetarians, and mixed peas, beans and lentils or quinoa for vegetarians. There is so much confusion about meat. Is it good or is it bad? This confusion arises because studies tend not to differentiate between types of meat. However, there is a big difference between grass-fed organic meat and processed meat like spam and sausages. When I first heard the term 'grass-fed cows', I thought it was a very odd phrase as I grew up on a Scottish island and thought that all cows were fed like that. Maybe we all picture cows roaming about the grass, chewing the cud quite happily. The reality is very different as most cows are now reared indoors and fed a cereal diet.

The fats of life: The importance of essential fatty acids

Have you been told that fats are bad and make you fat? Do you avoid fats but fill up with so-called 'healthy wholegrains' instead? These grains are not healthy at all but they are taking the place of more valuable foods. Of all the food we eat, the most confusion surrounds fats and oils. There are certain fats that we absolutely need, so much so that they are called *essential* fatty acids. We cannot make them in our bodies so we have to get them through our diet. These are called omega-3 and omega-6. I have devoted a whole section to this because the change in the types of fat eaten is very bad for our health.

Omega-3 and omega-6

We get our omega-3 from oily fish such as salmon, sardines, herring, anchovies and mackerel. Omega-6 comes from most fresh nuts and seeds such as flax, hemp, walnuts, sunflower seeds and pumpkin seeds, as well as corn. We need these very much but only in their natural state, as we did in times gone by. One study published in the *Scandinavian Journal of Epidemiology* compared levels of omega-3 in those with IBS and those without.[21] The IBS group was found to have lower levels, so try to make sure that you get your omegas right.

The problem is that, before food processing came about, we ate far less omega-6 and far more omega-3 than we do now. In the past, the ratio would have been 1:1 but now we consume twenty to forty times as much omega-6 as omega-3. Many of the health problems we suffer today are directly related to this imbalance. Now our bodies are full of the wrong oils for two reasons: firstly, we have too much omega-6 and secondly, that omega-6 is so highly processed that it does us no good at all.

Why not have processed oils?

In the past, we only had the oils that came from fish and whole nuts and seeds. We did not have these huge bottles of sunflower or other oils that we see today because we did not have the technology to extract them. Now just about everything in the supermarket is full of processed oil extracted from seeds (see the list overleaf). You can probably see why the ratio of omega-3 to omega-6 is so different to what it was. Processed oils are as nothing found in nature. One study found that those suffering from IBS had higher levels of arachidonic acid in their bodies. This is an omega-6 fat that causes inflammation.

Processed oils are everywhere

One problem with this is that we are now overloaded with omega-6 oils. The other problem is that these omega-6 oils are nearly always processed. This is bad because they cause inflammation, which is implicated in many diseases including bowel cancer, inflammatory bowel disease, heart disease and arthritis. Having learned how to extract oil from seeds using chemical solvents, manufacturers added them to just about everything. You will know that all fried foods contain them but so does just about every manufactured food in the super-market. This includes raisins! Oils are added to stop them sticking together.

Processed oil goes through so many processes (distilling, degumming, refining, bleaching and, because it smells so badly, deodorizing) that it ends up as something very dif-ferent from the nuts and seeds where it began. It is a huge amount of processing for a little sunflower seed.

Foods containing processed oils

- All fried foods including crisps, chips and battered fish
- All other savoury snacks
- Readymade soups
- Ready meals
- Pastries
- Cakes
- Most desserts
- Ice cream
- Biscuits
- Chocolate
- Dips
- Hummus, taramasalata

- Non-dairy creamer

- All oils except olive

- Margarine and other spreads

- Mayonnaise and other salad dressings

- Bread

- Some cereals

- Pies

- Quiche

- Samosas

- Sauces.

You might think by looking at this list that there is nothing left to eat. But it just shows you how much of these oils we are eating, often without realizing it. They are taking the place of the vegetables that we should be eating for the sake of our digestion and our health in general. This is why it is better to make food at home from scratch.

What happens after initial processing?

There is more to come. At this point, the oil is still liquid but in order to make it solid and look more like butter it is blasted with hydrogen atoms. This changes it yet again, making it into a trans-fat or hydrogenated fat. These are sold as spreads and margarines, and are considered so bad for you that many supermarkets in the UK have stopped selling them.

However, it is not just trans-fats that are bad: all processed oils, whether sunflower, soya or canola, are as bad as each other. It is best to avoid them at all costs. The problem is that supermarket shelves are full of products made from these oils. Everything that is fried contains them, as do most readymade foods such as soups, main meals, desserts and sauces (the list is endless). These fats and oils have been implicated in so many diseases that I urge you to keep away from them as much as possible.

If you are cooking, it is much better to use butter or coconut oil. It used to be thought that the saturated fat in these foods caused heart disease and that margarine was better. This is not the case. We have been eating saturated fat for most of our existence but heart disease is relatively new. Of course, butter is very high in calories and will increase weight if you eat too much of it, but it is a natural food.

Oils and inflammation

One of the problems of processed oils (there are many) is that they promote inflammation. On the other hand, omega-3 from fish reduces it. Inflammation is needed when we cut ourselves as it brings oxygen and nutrients to the site to help the wound heal. But too much chronic inflammation is bad and we need the anti-inflammatory effects of oily fish. However, processed oils compete with the omega-3 that we really need, so I recommend cutting them out of our diets entirely.

The oils that protect us

What should we be eating to get the oils we need? Firstly, we need omega-3 from oily fish: salmon (organic), mackerel, herring and sardines are good but tuna is a large fish and can contain too much mercury. Smaller fish are better. Omega-3 helps to prevent all sorts of diseases including heart disease, cancer, arthritis, brain deterioration and more.

Vegetarians can get good oils from flaxseeds and walnut but these need to be converted in the body to the docosahexaenoic acid (DHA) and eicosapentaenoic acid (EPA) found in oily fish. Not everyone can make this conversion easily.

Increasing your vitamin D intake

Do you remember being given cod liver oil as a child? This was given as a good source of vitamin D3 and many of us had to have teaspoons of this fishy-tasting product to help prevent rickets or bent bones. Later on, vitamin D drops were given to children and still are today. Strangely enough, vitamin D is not really a vitamin at all. It is actually a steroid hormone, which is needed to absorb various nutrients.

Research is now showing that low levels of vitamin D are associated with higher levels of IBS. In one study, people with IBS were compared to a matched group with normal digestion (the control group).[22] Of those, only 32 per cent of the control group had low levels of vitamin D but a massive 82 per cent of the IBS group were deficient. Another study

IDEAS FOR MEALS

PROTEIN	VEGETABLES	FATS	OTHER
Choose One	Choose Three	Choose One	Additional
Chicken	Carrots	1 teaspoon extra virgin olive oil	Potatoes
Sardines (fresh or in water)	Sweet potatoes		Rice
Turkey	Peas	2 teaspoons butter	Fruit
Cod (not fried)	Courgettes		
Mackerel	Green beans	1 tablespoon flaxseeds	
Herring	Lettuce	Handful walnuts	
Lean meat (organic)	Tomatoes		
2 eggs (organic)	Cucumber	Sesame, sunflower seeds	
Quinoa	Celery		
Haddock (not fried)	Fennel	Seeds and fruit can be eaten as snacks	
Salmon (organic)	Cauliflower		
Mix of peas, beans and lentils	Broccoli	(No salted or roasted nuts)	
	Cabbage		
	Parsnips		
	Swede		
	Other vegetables		

published in the *British Medical Journal* found that high-dose supplementation of vitamin D helped 70 per cent of those studied.

Nowadays this vitamin seems to be all over the news. In fact, one doctor has said that in his entire career he has never known a substance get the media attention that vitamin D is getting today. Reports keep coming in that people living in colder climates and even some in hotter climates are not getting enough. This is because vitamin D is made from sunlight interacting with the oils on our skin but we tend to protect ourselves with sun creams and clothes (and women wear trousers more often now). On top of this, even when we do sunbathe we often shower or bathe once or twice a day, which washes the oil from our skin and prevents the manufacture of vitamin D.

Certain people are more likely than others to be deficient in vitamin D: those with darker skins, older adults and those who are overweight. Very few foods contain it naturally, although it has been added to some so our main sources are sunlight and supplements.

We do need to get some sun but be very careful not to burn, especially as the incidents of skin cancer are rising. It is better to keep away from the midday sun and to wear sun lotion, a hat and sunglasses. If you choose to sit in the sun with arms and legs exposed and your face covered up, you can still get enough vitamin D. Why get wrinkles if you can avoid it?

Test for low vitamin D

As low levels of vitamin D are implicated in so many conditions it is important for all of us to have this checked even if we don't have IBS. It is a simple blood test and easy to get on the NHS. If levels are low, you can take supplements along with getting some sun (if possible), and then retest a few months later.

The importance of water

Did you know that we are 70 per cent water? Are you drinking enough? It is very important for your digestion that you do as your body's water needs to be replenished throughout the day.

Many people, especially older people who often don't feel thirsty even when they need water, are dehydrated without realizing it. I have known of people who drink nothing but tea and coffee with just the odd glass of water here and there. Tea and coffee are not terrible but they are not great for hydration either (green tea is very beneficial, however) so water is needed in addition to these. We should aim to drink about eight glasses a day, and more on a hot day.

Be careful about the water that you drink. Tap water is not the water we would have drunk in the natural state: water companies remove some impurities but do not remove all the chemicals. It is often contaminated with hormone-type chemicals and other drugs and, in addition, chemicals like chlorine and aluminium are added to the water in an attempt to purify it!

Bottled water

This is not always what it seems. Some bottled waters are just filtered tap water. Check the label for the words 'natural mineral water', which means that it has come from an officially registered source.

Although bottled water can be a good alternative to tap water, it is not a good idea to buy it in plastic containers. This is because chemicals from plastic can leach into the water. One quite common chemical called Bisphenol A (BPA) is implicated in breast cancer. So if you do buy bottled water, try to get it in glass bottles even though it is more expensive and the bottles are heavier than plastic. If you are out and need to buy water in a plastic bottle, keep it cool and don't leave it in the sun as heat causes more chemicals to leach into the water.

Filtered water

It is a good idea to filter tap water for drinking or soups because it contains so many chemicals. The simplest method for filtering water is to have a jug with a carbon filter attached to it: just pour the water into the jug and pour it out through the filter. The filter needs to be changed regularly. There are other, more sophisticated filters and water purifiers that have to be plumbed into your house. Some can also clean the water that you use for washing and bathing. These are good because they prevent us from lying in water that contains toxins. Some think that reverse osmosis filters are the best but they do contain some plastic.

The FODMAP diet

This particular diet has become quite popular in recent years. It involves cutting out very many nutritious foods that some people find difficult to digest. It is not a cure and does not get to the underlying *cause* of the condition but some people seem to feel better on it.

In my opinion it is a bit like saying, 'My knee hurts when I go upstairs', and your friend says, 'Well, don't go upstairs.' This misses the point. The point is that you *should* be able to digest most common foods, and you need to find out *why* you can't digest them. It may be that you lack digestive enzymes or have candida.

Some of the foods that the FODMAP diet cuts out are highly nutritious and some such as broccoli and cabbage are even cancer protective. It is not a good idea to cut out so many highly nutritious foods, except in the very short term. I think it is far better to strengthen your digestive system so that you *can* eat these foods. However, if you are interested in reading about the FODMAP diet, there are many books on the subject.

In a nutshell

- To have good digestion we need to eat as nature intended, which means eating foods that are fresh, unprocessed and free from artificial additives.

- The most important foods are vegetables as these contain the greatest amount of vitamins, minerals and phytochemicals. Eat a rainbow of coloured fruits and vegetables.

- Other foods to include are organic eggs, meat and chicken, nuts and seeds (ground for poor digestion), millet, quinoa and yogurt (perhaps made from coconut milk).

- We should not have any processed oils, such as sunflower oil or margarine, or foods made from them.

- We should try to cook food from scratch as much as possible.

Chapter 8

DEALING WITH INDIVIDUAL CONDITIONS

People who have been diagnosed with IBS have many symptoms that warrant this diagnosis. However, there are many others who do not have IBS but still suffer from digestive problems like constipation or heartburn. This section deals with these. Of course if you do have IBS the information below will also be useful for you.

Constipation

Do you sometimes dread going to the toilet? Are your motions hard and difficult to pass? Does passing them cause pain and discomfort? Do you have less than one bowel movement a day? Many people who do not have IBS have constant or intermittent constipation and this can cause a fair amount of discomfort and even pain when trying to pass solid, hard stools. The problem is that we don't often talk about these things so many people might not know what a normal motion should look like.

Charts have been drawn up describing different kinds

of bowel movements ranging from pellets to very watery loose diarrhoea. The ideal would be a stool that looked like a brown banana and was easy to pass without straining or pain. There should be no bits of undigested food in it and it should break up in the water of the toilet.

It is amazing how many people suffer from digestive problems but accept them as normal. For example, passing a motion every three days might be the norm for some but it is still constipation even if it is easy to pass. You really need to have a motion at least once a day.

Long-term constipation is not good because it can lead to other, more serious conditions. It can cause haemorrhoids (piles), varicose veins in the legs and diverticulitis, where the colon bulges out into little pockets. Piles are bulging veins in the rectum like varicose veins in the legs. They can itch, bleed and become painful. If you do suffer from piles, the first thing to do is to try to make your stools looser.

Causes of constipation

Constipation is very common and when it occurs, many turn to over-the-counter medications to help deal with it. These can be used in the very short term but it is much better to find the underlying cause and deal with that. Using medication in the long term can make the situation worse and it is therefore important to get your system working naturally. Constipation can be caused by:

- dehydration or not drinking enough;
- lack of fibre;
- low levels of magnesium;
- low thyroid;
- not exercising enough;
- not enough good bacteria;
- poor diet in general.

Dehydration: are you drinking enough?

Do you sometimes forget to drink? Are you often just too busy to stop? Do you go for long periods on coffee but no water? I hope not because this will cause dry, hard stools that are difficult to pass. It is important to have enough water in your system to make your stools soft and bulky. It is vital to drink water in particular as it is best for hydrating the body while tea and coffee can be dehydrating. We need about eight glasses of good water a day and more on a hot day or if you are exercising and sweating a lot. Tea and coffee might appear to be adding fluids, but don't rely on them alone. On the other hand, green tea has many health benefits but drink it in addition to water rather than instead of it. It is a good idea to sip water throughout the day rather than ingest large amounts all at once.

Not eating enough fibre

See Chapter 4 for details about this.

Low levels of magnesium

If you are not only constipated but are also suffering from fatigue, high blood pressure or anxiety, you may be lacking in magnesium. Magnesium is a mineral that helps us relax, builds bones, helps us sleep and has many other functions in the body. One important thing that it does for digestion is that it keeps stools soft. In fact, if you have too much magnesium it can cause diarrhoea. However, many of us in the West are deficient in magnesium because the processed foods sold in supermarkets contain very little. A study published in the *European Journal of Clinical Nutrition* supports this.[23]

The problem is that even foods such as green vegetables that should contain magnesium will not contain much if the soil in which they are grown is deficient. Poor farming practices do not help, as farmers often do not replace this mineral. If a mineral is not there in the soil, it cannot get into the food grown on it and so it cannot get into us.

Too much calcium in relation to magnesium

Another reason why we tend to be low in magnesium is that it needs to be balanced with calcium. Too much calcium can cause a deficiency of magnesium. You might wonder how you can have too much calcium as this is often thought to be so important in preventing bone diseases like osteoporosis. The reason is that we as a nation eat huge amounts of calcium in all sorts of foods. Think about all the calcium-rich foods available in the shops: all the dairy products such as milk, yogurt and fromage frais, so many different cheeses, cheese added to foods like pizza, cheese sauce, cheesecake, ice cream, milky desserts, buttermilk and more. You can see, therefore, how easy it is to ingest lots of calcium.

On the other hand, magnesium is found mainly in green leafy vegetables, nuts and seeds. These foods are eaten much less often than all the milky foods and there are so few of them anyway that we are more likely to be deficient in magnesium.

In addition to this, there are foods that actually rob the body of magnesium. These are oxalates in spinach and rhubarb, and phytates in wheat bran and wholemeal breads. All these high-fibre, wheat-based cereals are not helping our levels of magnesium.

Symptoms of magnesium deficiency

Magnesium helps us relax and when we don't have enough we get symptoms of agitation. Other symptoms are muscle weakness, insomnia, nervousness, constipation, calcium deposits in soft tissue and high blood pressure. These, of course, can also be caused by other factors.

As magnesium has so many functions in the body, it is a good idea to have a test for a deficiency. It is important that the test carried out is for red cell magnesium. You can have this tested via your doctor but, if this is not possible, a nutritional therapist can arrange it for you using a private laboratory.

Foods high in magnesium

- Green leafy vegetables
- Almonds
- Cashew nuts
- Brazil nuts
- Pecan nuts
- Cooked beans (soak first)
- Bananas.

Although nuts are good sources of magnesium, many people with digestive problems find them difficult to digest. Grind them first or stick to green vegetables until you feel better.

Are you eating enough healthy fat?

Despite their bad press, fats are needed in the diet and perform many functions, one of which is to keep the digestive tract lubricated (see Chapter 7 on 'The fats of life'). Examples of good fats are avocadoes, ground flaxseeds, coconut oil, egg yolks, organic butter, oily fish and organic meat. Very low-fat diets are not a good idea.

Exercise

This can help constipation by massaging the intestines. One study of Chinese adolescents found that constipation was associated with lack of exercise. Exercise is good for just about everything as well as refreshing sleep and reducing stress. The form of exercise does not really matter so do something that you enjoy. The days of 'no pain, no gain' are over and ordinary walking in your daily life can help quite a lot.

Low levels of thyroid hormone

The thyroid is the gland that controls metabolism. It produces the hormone thyroxine and if we do not have enough, we become slow and sluggish and so does our digestive system. However, the good news is that an underactive thyroid is very easy to test and treat. If you have other symptoms related to this, such as feeling cold all the time, weight gain, fatigue, thinning hair and eyebrows, dry skin, and muscle and joint pains, ask your doctor to test you for this. It involves just a simple blood test. If you are found to be low in thyroxine, it can be easily treated.

It is interesting that some people who are technically within the normal range can still be low in thyroxine compared to others. For example, if the normal range of thyroxine is 11 to 28 and your level is 12, you might be in the normal range but you still only have half as much as someone with a level of 24. So discuss your levels with your doctor along with your symptoms.

Probiotics

Again, these are important (see Chapter 5). One study published in the *Turkish Journal of Gastroenterology* found that kefir improved stool frequency and also improved scores of bowel satisfaction.[23]

Coeliac disease

All sufferers of digestive problems should be tested for coeliac disease, and it involves just a simple blood test. It is important to rule this out because it could be causing your symptoms and needs to be dealt with as soon as possible. Most of the conditions in this book do not involve damage to the lining of the gut but coeliac disease, which does cause damage, needs to be ruled out.

What is coeliac disease?

In our digestive tract, we have villi, which are tiny hairs. At first glance they look like a brush and are sometimes referred to as the brush border. Their function is to increase the surface area where food can be absorbed. The problem is that when some people eat gluten (which is found in grains, mainly wheat) it causes the villi to wear away, leaving a smooth surface. The absence of villi prevents food being digested properly, which causes chronic diarrhoea. This in turn results in nutrients not being absorbed properly. The main symptoms are:

- diarrhoea (the principal symptom);
- bloating;
- gas;
- fluid retention;

- malnutrition from not digesting food properly for a sustained period.

The good news

Coeliac disease is not an allergy as such but an autoimmune disease where the body attacks itself. Fortunately, this disease is easy to treat and when gluten grains are excluded from the diet, the villi grow back again. The person remains healthy as long as gluten is kept out of the diet. It is as easy as that. On the other hand, people with this condition need to cut out foods containing gluten forever. This can be difficult for some as it is contained in many foods that you might not suspect, such as salad dressings and ice cream. However, while it can take some time to get used to, it is better for our health overall to eat fresh, natural, home-cooked food. There are also many gluten-free products now widely available but they are not very nutritious. However, you might like to use them occasionally.

As we discussed earlier, many people don't have coeliac disease but still cannot tolerate wheat very well. In any case, some nutritionists say that wheat is not a good food for anyone. The fact that coeliac disease exists shows how damaging wheat can be for some people.

Test for coeliac disease

If you suspect that you might have coeliac disease, you will need to have a test carried out by your GP. However, it is probably a good idea for all IBS sufferers to have this test. The test is not difficult and just involves looking for antibodies to gluten in the blood plus transglutaminase and endomysial antibodies. The test is 99 per cent accurate. You should not give up gluten before having the test because this in itself will stop the production of antibodies, which will make the test invalid. If you are found to have this condition, you need to work with your doctor.

Helicobacter pylori infection

This is not really a condition but a tongue-twisting name for a very dangerous bacterium! However, *Helicobacter pylori* (*H. pylori*) is a nuisance that is able to contaminate our foods and water supplies. It can reside in the stomach and cause many mild and some serious problems. For example, it can cause or mimic acid indigestion and gastritis, and is often the culprit behind the formation of stomach ulcers. It can even go on to cause stomach cancer so it is important to rule it out.

Infection with *H. pylori* is so common that it affects about half of the world's population. One American study found that more than 60 per cent of those over sixty had it and it is estimated that about 40 per cent of UK citizens have it and up to 50 per cent of the world's population are sufferers. It has even been discovered in household cats!

The discovery of H. pylori

There is an interesting story attached to *H. pylori*. It was first discovered by the Australian doctor Barry Marshall in the early 1980s. At the time, everyone thought that ulcers were caused by too much acid in the stomach or being over-stressed. Marshall thought instead that it was caused by some sort of bacterium. Other doctors and practitioners apparently ridiculed him for this because they thought that bacteria could not survive for long in the highly acidic stomach. In fact, one of the functions of stomach acid is to kill any bad bacteria that we ingest.

Consequently, Marshall was ignored for about ten years. However, he knew he was right so to prove it he cultured the bacterium and drank it himself. He promptly got gastritis (inflammation of the stomach). This led to his ideas being looked at again and it is now accepted that he was right. *H. pylori* does cause ulcers and worse, and now doctors look for it as a matter of routine if these are present. To add to his vindication, Barry Marshall and J. Robin Warren were awarded the Nobel Prize in 2005 for their work on *H. pylori*.

A very clever bacterium

H. pylori can survive in the strong acid of the stomach because it has an unusual helical shape, which allows it to burrow into the stomach wall like a corkscrew. What it does next is very clever. It produces its own alkalis to neutralize the stomach acid around it, which means that there is less acid left to kill the bacterium itself. Very smart! This is an example of how we are in a constant battle with organisms in the environment. The good news, however, is that *H. pylori* is very easy to treat with medication or natural substances.

H. pylori does not only affect the stomach. It can also affect other parts of the body and has also been implicated in other diseases. Examples are Parkinson's, psoriasis, autoimmune conditions such as thyroiditis and Sjögren's syndrome. This is because it can make the gut leaky (see Chapter 6).

As mentioned, many people who have acid reflux or heartburn now buy antacids over the counter or get them on prescription. Although these can help relieve the symptoms in the long run they cause other problems because they take away stomach acid (see Chapter 4). We need stomach acid in order to kill bugs such as *H. pylori* and to break up protein foods like meat, eggs and fish.

Symptoms of H. pylori infection

- Excessive burping
- Feeling bloated
- Nausea and vomiting
- Abdominal discomfort

On the other hand, some infected people have no symptoms.

Test for H. pylori

This can be carried out by your GP. The best test is a breath test. If you have this bacterium in your stomach, your breath will show the presence of ammonia and carbon dioxide. It is a simple test in which you give two breath samples after fasting for six hours.

Treatment

The usual medical treatment for *H. pylori* is two types of antibiotics plus a proton pump inhibitor that stops acid for two weeks. However, one doctor, Dr Sherry Rogers, advises that this can be very harsh.[25] She recommends Pepto-Bismol, which can be bought over the counter, but you should discuss this with your doctor first.

Additional help for prevention

*   *Green tea*: this can help slow down the growth of *H. pylori*. Green tea is a very valuable drink in many ways and it even has anti-cancer and anti-inflammatory properties. It is a good idea to try to get organic green tea as some non-organic versions have been found to contain DDT from pesticides.

*   *Garlic*: this amazingly beneficial food is also anti-viral, anti-fungal and anti-antiseptic, and helps thin the blood.

*   *Turmeric*: this can also be helpful in killing *H. pylori*.

*   *Vitamin C*: this has also been shown to help prevent *H. pylori* infection.

Haemorrhoids

This is a very common problem related to our digestion. It

means that the veins near the anus, either inside or outside, are dilated or blown out like varicose veins. Although they are not dangerous, they can be very painful and uncomfortable. If they bleed, the blood tends to be bright red. Any bleeding should be checked out by your doctor in order to rule out conditions that are more serious.

They sometimes begin in pregnancy or during childbirth because at this time more pressure is put on the veins, but generally haemorrhoids or piles are usually caused by constipation. When we press down, trying to pass a hard stool, this puts pressure on the veins, making them bulge out. Passing hard stools past haemorrhoids can be extremely painful so it is very important to avoid constipation and keep the stools soft. Haemorrhoids can't really be cured but if the stools are kept soft and easy to pass then they should not cause any problems. The diet recommended for constipation described earlier should help.

Haemorrhoids can also be caused by a deficiency of magnesium, which is very common in Western countries because of food processing. Magnesium helps muscles to relax and this includes the muscles in the digestive system. Be careful not to take too much as this can have the opposite effect and cause loose stools (keep to the instructions on the bottle).

Help for haemorrhoids

- Bathing the area in cold water every morning can help.

- Suppositories from the chemist can help but be careful if there is a tear as this can cause itching and pain (do not use them if your skin is sensitive).

- The food supplement Pycnogenol taken orally and as a topical treatment has been shown to help.

- It is better to try to squat than sit while passing a motion. Sitting puts the wrong sort of pressure on our veins and, until recent times, we would have squatted when emptying our bowels.

- Herbs such as horse chestnut or butcher's broom can help strengthen and tone veins.

- Sitz baths: sit in three to four inches of warm water in a bath for ten minutes several times a day; a quarter cup of Epsom salts can be added.

- If your anus itches and becomes irritated, it may be due to the paper. Some papers are less irritating than others and some health-food shops sell unbleached paper.

Diarrhoea

You have probably suffered from this from time to time as most of us have. It is not a disease but a symptom and it can have many causes. It is your body's attempt to get rid of what it does not like. However, although we all get this occasionally it is not normal to have chronic diarrhoea. If it is severe, especially in babies and children, it needs to be treated very quickly and they should be seen by a doctor right away.

If you have chronic diarrhoea, your food is not being digested properly: it is going through your system too quickly and you are not getting the benefit of it. During a bout, you need to drink lots of fluids in order to stay hydrated. Vegetable juices and broths are a good idea as they provide some nutrition as well.

If you have a new bout of this condition, think back to what you have been doing. Have you been on holiday? Perhaps you have picked up a parasite. What did you eat the day before? Did you eat out? Did you have any unusual foods? Have you been under more stress?

If the condition is chronic then you need to find the underlying cause. The ideas in this book should help overall but specifically the cause could be diverticular disease, infections, parasites, IBS, IBD, candida, lactose intolerance or even cancer. The following tests are available.

- Comprehensive digestive stool analysis with a parasite test, usually carried out in private laboratories. You can have this done through a qualified nutritionist.

- SIBO–hydrogen breath test.

- Lactose breath test

- Allergy or food intolerance tests.

Help for diarrhoea

- In the short term, you can buy sachets of electrolytes from the chemist.

- Drink plenty of fluids to avoid dehydration (broths are good).

- Keep your hands very clean, especially when preparing food.

- Take the probiotic *Saccharomyces boulardii*, which increases secretory IgA and can help prevent and treat diarrhoea caused by travel or antibiotics.

- Take other probiotics.

- Fibre such as psyllium can help make the stool more solid as it absorbs the liquid.

- If it persists, visit your GP.

Diverticular disease

Unlike IBS, this condition *does* involve physical changes of the colon. I have included it here because it is very common but quite easy to relieve with the right diet. Diverticular disease is where pea-sized pouches, called diverticula, bulge out of the wall of the colon. It is often caused by constipation because the colon finds it difficult to pass along dry, hard faecal matter. The extra pressure causes the bowel to blow or bulge out over time. The problem is that bits of food can fall into these pouches and become trapped there. Often there are no symptoms but, in other cases, the pouches can become infected, irritated and inflamed, causing pain and fever. This is called diverticulitis, which means inflammation of the diverticula.

Treatment

When this happens, antibiotics are needed to treat the infection. The diverticula never go away but the right diet can stop food dropping into these pouches and causing problems. The diet needs to be one that prevents constipation and is made up of foods that are smooth, soft and bulky. Foods that have small particles like seeds, nuts and even partly chewed crisps or corn flakes should be avoided as these can easily drop into the pouches. If you eat soft, well-cooked vegetables, blended soups and other mushy foods, they will pass along the digestive tract more easily. Potatoes and mashed root vegetables can be quite soothing. You also need to eat protein foods for healing and these should be easy to digest. Scrambled eggs and fish are good suggestions.

When the infection has been treated, you need to take steps to heal the lining of your digestive tract. This can be done with:

- aloe vera;
- gamma oryzanol;
- *Lactobacillus acidophilus/Bifidobacterium*;
- bone broths.

Heartburn

If you have ever suffered from heartburn, you will know that it can be very unpleasant and worrying. It is painful and makes us want to reach for an antacid right away. The acid in our stomach is very strong but it needs to be in order to help digest our food properly and kill off unwanted bacteria. However, it should stay where it's meant to be, in the stomach. When it escapes from the stomach and travels up into the oesophagus, this is felt as heartburn. We can suffer from this because the sphincter at the top of the stomach, which keeps the acid in place, weakens and the acid can easily back up into the oesophagus. This can cause belching and burping after meals and a feeling of burning above the stomach.

Of course, burping and belching can be caused simply by swallowing air or drinking fizzy drinks. However, if it feels acidic and painful, it could well be caused by something more.

It is because of heartburn that many people take antacids, but while these are fine for the odd occasion, they are not meant to be used long term because we really need our stomach acid (see Chapter 4).

If you belch and burp a lot, the first thing you should do is to be tested for the bacterium *Helicobacter pylori* discussed earlier. This bug can live in the stomach and cause stomach ulcers or even stomach cancer. A simple test can be carried out by your GP and it can be eradicated with either antibiotics or natural supplements.

Gastroesophageal reflux disease (GERD)

This is the same as heartburn and acid reflux. One cause is a hiatus hernia, which means that part of the stomach bulges through a little opening called a hiatus. Another cause is stress or anxiety, which you should try to reduce. This is not always easy but see Chapter 10 for some ideas.

Do you love spicy food? If you do and are getting acid reflux, this could be a contributor. Other foods that can be a problem are orange juice, tomatoes, mint, coffee, fried foods and chocolate. Some medications can also cause GERD so it is a good idea to check these with your doctor.

Flatulence and wind

Do you ever feel that your stomach is all blown up? Do your skirts or trousers often feel tight? Do you often prefer to wear elastic waistbands at these times? Does your stomach sometimes look as if you are pregnant and then flatten again a few days later? The programme outlined in this book should help with this. In particular, clearing candida, helping constipation and making the whole system work better should make frequent wind problems a thing of the past. However, below are some extra ideas for beating the bloat.

We all know how embarrassing wind can be, especially when we are in company. Actually, it is normal to pass wind or gas about ten to fifteen times a day because we tend to swallow air when eating. However, if we have too much we tend to blow up like a balloon and this makes us feel bloated and uncomfortable. In fact, not passing it can feel worse than passing it because trapped wind is extremely uncomfortable.

Not all gas smells bad. The type that does comes from eating foods rich in the mineral sulphur. You may be familiar with the smell of rotten eggs.

Causes of flatulence

There are many causes and some of these are listed below. Generally, the cause is poorly digested food fermenting in the gut.

- Swallowing air while eating.
- Undigested food that ferments in the digestive tract.
- Yeast overgrowth.
- Low levels of stomach acid and/or digestive enzymes, which means that food is not being digested properly.
- Lactose intolerance.

For those who have very bad gas on the odd occasion without other symptoms the following ideas should help.

Help for flatulence

- Ginger tea made with fresh ginger can sometimes help expel the gas. Grate some ginger into boiled water and drink. You can also use teabags or a half-teaspoon of ginger powder in a cup of boiled water. Incidentally, ginger also relieves the nausea of pregnancy.
- Chewing fennel seeds can help. These can be found in

the spices area of the supermarket. They have a very pleasant taste like aniseed. Sometimes they are given out after meals in Indian restaurants.

- Activated charcoal tablets can bring relief. These can also make your stools black so don't be alarmed.

- Try digestive enzymes such as bromelain, papaya or pancreatic enzymes.

- Peppermint oil capsules can also help, as can peppermint tea.

- Kneeling on the floor with your bottom in the air can sometimes help.

Preventing flatulence

- Eat regular meals and sit down to eat.

- Chew all food well. This is very important for carbohydrate foods such as potatoes, which will ferment if not properly mixed with saliva.

- Don't eat under stressful conditions or 'on the run'.

- Test for lactose intolerance and if needed, deal with that.

- Try avoiding soy sauce, cheese and alcohol.

- Try not to eat fried foods, which are harmful in many ways.

- Fruit should be eaten alone as it can ferment in the digestive tract if eaten with other foods (melon can be particularly bad in this respect).

- If you eat beans, soak them for 4–12 hours, drain off the water and cook them in fresh water.

- Some people cannot tolerate apple, cabbage, cucumber, onion, chickpeas, lentils and other pulses.

- Vitamin B5 has been shown to relieve intestinal gas and distension. Take as part of a multi-vitamin/mineral supplement.

- Try cleansing the colon with Lepicol psyllium husks: this 'sweeps up' undigested fibrous material left fermenting in the colon. You need two teaspoons morning and evening in a large glass of water, and should drink a second glass of water with it to prevent any constipation getting worse. You may need a smaller dose to begin with in order to get used to it.

Chapter 9

HOW TO EAT FOR GOOD DIGESTION

Have you ever seen early TV dramas where everyone is sitting down quietly around the table eating their meal? It is often very calm and still, and sometimes all you can hear is a clock ticking loudly as family members slurp their soup. Usually everyone seems relaxed, eating slowly and there is no tension. It all looks a little artificial by today's standards but this way of eating supports good digestion. Nowadays there is often lots of noise, bustle and argument while we eat so it is almost impossible to digest our food completely.

What you eat is very important but *how* you eat matters tremendously. It makes a huge difference to your ability to digest your food properly. So often, we are eating while doing something else like working, arguing, sitting in a train or even walking in the street.

Are you eating under stress?

Are you eating your breakfast while putting on your coat or running out of the door? Do you eat lunch at your desk while answering phones or talking to colleagues? Do you run about the house or the streets with a sandwich in your hand?

Perhaps you are a mum who gets up and down all through the meal to serve or to get things for the others. Are you serving and eating at the same time? Alternatively, are you trying to eat your food while cutting up your children's food or trying to spoon food into tiny mouths? Are you eating your own food while worrying about what your kids are eating or, more likely, what they will *not* eat?

Many children are fussy eaters, making their mums tense and nervous at the table. Maybe you are not a mum but a slimmer worrying about what *you* are eating. Is it too high in calories? Is it making you fat?

All of these situations hinder proper digestion. One of my clients came to me very distressed about her indigestion, wind and bloating, especially in the afternoons. On questioning, I soon discovered that she ate her lunch at her work desk, talking to people on the phone, answering queries from colleagues and so on. I advised her to take a proper lunch break and go into another room to read a magazine or go out and sit in a park. This was all it took for her problems to clear up. Of course, it may not be as simple as this for everyone but, whatever else you do, try not to eat under stress.

Avoiding drinking while eating

Do you like to have a nice cup of tea with your meals? I know I do. We tend to eat and drink at the same time and take it for granted that we should. Usually we have our tea, coffee or water with a meal and see that as the natural thing to do. However, drinking and eating at the same time can affect our digestion quite badly so try to wait about half an hour after eating before having a drink. Drinking while eating can dilute the much-needed enzymes in your saliva and your stomach acid, which is not good because these are needed to help break down your food.

It is also good to eat little and often rather than eating large meals all at once. Small meals every three hours should keep your blood sugar stable and prevent you from getting too hungry. If we allow ourselves to become too hungry, we are much more likely to gulp food down quickly without chewing it properly. So don't leave it too long before having something to eat.

Getting your digestive juices flowing

Where does digestion start?

You might think that digestion begins in the stomach or even in the mouth but really neither is true: it begins in the brain. Try thinking about your favourite food or even go into your kitchen and have a look at it. Can you feel your mouth watering? If so, this is your glands producing the saliva needed to digest the food. Even if you can't detect the saliva, it is still there, ready and waiting. When the saliva is produced, other things start to happen in your body. Your stomach starts producing hydrochloric acid in anticipation, blood flow is diverted away from your limbs to your stomach and your whole system prepares for the food. Blood going to your limbs is less important at this time because your body is not expecting to eat and run.

Tempting smells

When you enter a supermarket, do you often crave bread? That is because the smell of it frequently pervades the whole place. We know that even the smell, look and thought of food make things happen in our bodies. Foods that look and smell good help to get our digestive fluids flowing. We look forward to eating our favourite foods and foods that we don't like the look of can hinder digestion. Even some animals smell food before deciding whether to eat it.

Once we have put the food into our mouths this starts the next stage in our digestion.

The importance of chewing

Our mothers were right when they told us to chew our food well but when we are in a hurry, we often forget. This is not good because digestion starts in the mouth and we need to chew so that our food can mix with saliva. Our saliva contains enzymes, which help us digest certain foods so this is important. The enzymes in saliva are called amylase and these help digest carbohydrate foods like bread, potatoes, fruits and vegetables. The food is then acted on by enzymes secreted from the pancreas in order to break it down further. As well as amylase, they include protease to break down protein like meat, eggs and fish, and lipase to break down fats. Because chewing is so vital for good digestion, don't wait to eat until you are too hungry. You might then swallow anything that is not nailed down just to feel better, or gulp it down too quickly. This could mean that large lumps of food end up sitting unchewed in your stomach. When we chew our food, we digest it better so try to wait until it becomes a soft mush before swallowing it. Here, then, is another reason to eat when you need to and have regular meal times.

Not chewing causes wind

Chewing grinds the food into a paste. If food is not properly chewed, it reaches the small intestine in the wrong form and this can cause wind, bloating and cramping. I hope, therefore, that I have convinced you not to let your food leave your mouth too soon.

Be careful when liquidizing whole raw vegetables in powerful blenders, which have become so popular. Although these machines are very valuable and allow you to consume lots of raw food, and literally drink your vegetables, you still need to coat them in saliva. So if you have one try to swill the liquid around in your mouth before swallowing. The carbohydrate in it still needs to mix with the amylase in your saliva.

After we swallow, the food hits our stomach and then the very powerful stomach acid breaks it down. This is so important for good digestion that I have devoted a whole section to it (see Chapter 4). After eating, sit down quietly and let the food be digested. Getting up from the table and rushing around too soon is as bad as not sitting down at all.

Fibrous foods

Chewing well is especially important when we eat foods that are difficult to break down. Foods like raw vegetables, nuts and seeds can be difficult to digest because they are hard and fibrous. In fact, it might actually be better to stay away from foods like raw carrots and raw celery until you feel better, and nuts in particular are extremely challenging for some people. You might need to grind or soak them beforehand. In any case, we need to chew foods like this especially carefully. This may be obvious, but what is less obvious is that soft and mushy foods need to be well chewed too. Although these do not appear to need breaking down they still need to be mixed with the digestive enzymes in our saliva. Try to savour your food and really enjoy every bite. Think about what you are eating while you are doing it rather than eating while doing something else.

In a nutshell

- Try not to eat on the run. Sit down to quietly enjoy and savour your food.

- Eat little and often rather than having very large meals.

- Try not to have arguments at the table.

- Stay at the table for a while after eating.

- When at work leave your desk and eat quietly somewhere else.

- Chew, chew and chew your food thoroughly.

- Wait about half an hour before drinking.

- Relax and think pleasant thoughts while eating.

Chapter 10

STRESS AND DIGESTION

Stress and IBS definitely go hand in hand or, to be more specific, it is the anxiety caused by stress that affects us. Stress is part of life but, if you have a very stressful lifestyle, this could be affecting your digestion. I know that often we don't have control over our stress levels so it always amuses me when we are told to reduce them. If only it was so easy. We don't choose to have the challenges that we have, but if we can do something about them, our digestion will thank us for it.

We should try not to eat when under stress as it can fuel IBS and other digestive problems. Our minds and our bodies are not separate from each other: they are interconnected. For example, hormones can cause depression in women before a period and during the menopause. On the other hand, worry, stress and negative thoughts can affect our immune systems and cause physical illness. Stress can lower the natural killer cells in our bodies. These are important because they seek out and destroy viruses and other harmful cells. In fact, research has shown that cancer can often attack after a very stressful event. Long-term stress can have a damaging effect but even short-term stress can cause problems, too.

Understanding the link between stress and good digestion

The stress response

You must have felt the stress response many times. Perhaps you have had to speak in public or sit in a dentist's waiting room waiting for treatment. You might feel your heart beat faster, your muscles tighten and your mouth going dry. On the other hand, you may not realize that your blood pressure has shot up, sugar is mobilized into your bloodstream and your digestive system has shut down. All of these responses prepare us to either run away from the danger or fight it. In primitive times when we ventured out of our cave, we might come across a sabre-toothed tiger. We would then have to fight or run, which is why stress response is called the 'fight or flight' response. However, nowadays our stressors are different (they are not sabre-toothed tigers but deadlines, mortgages, screaming children, or arguments) but the stress response is just the same.

Happy stress

An odd thing about stress is that it works in the same way whatever the stress might be. For example, we know that dangerous and fearful situations can trigger it, but so can happy and exciting things. Your heart races and you have more energy when in danger or frightened, but it can also race when you experience good things. We would call this excitement rather than stress but the response is similar. Even

151

when excited in a good way, all the same arousal factors start to come into play. Our energy increases, our heart races, our digestion slows down and we can then start running to the toilet more often. Situations like being offered a promotion or having a party can cause it, and often brides say that they were too excited to eat anything at their own wedding. Of course, this will vary according to your own personality as some people are more excitable than others are.

Whatever the stress, part of the stress response is to slow down or shut down the digestive process. This makes sense because, when in danger, we need to use all our resources to fight or run away. There is no need to digest food at that time. This is all perfectly reasonable but the problem is that, because of our modern lifestyle, we still eat when under stress. We may be at our desk at work eating our lunch while operating the phones or grabbing a sandwich at the station. This is not conducive to good digestion.

If you have been in a stressful situation it is better to relax first, calm down and then eat. Eating immediately when you come home from work, having battled the Underground or traffic jams, is not good for digestion even though you may be starving. Wait a while until you are more relaxed and your food will be better digested.

Stress and IBS

Some studies show that IBS is very much affected by stress. One study published in the medical journal *Gastroenterology* stated that, 'There is strong evidence to support that IBS is a stress-sensitive disorder.'[26] It is becoming clear that what happens in our minds affects the rest of our body and that what we feel affects our gut. This is referred to as 'gut-brain interaction'. A study in the *World Journal of Gastroenterology* claimed that, 'More and more clinical and experimental evidence showed that IBS is a combination of irritable bowel and irritable brain'.[27] So attempting to lower our stress levels should go some way towards helping digestive problems.

Stress hormones

So what makes these stress responses happen? The two chemicals that do this are the hormones adrenaline and cortisol. Adrenaline is responsible for the fight or flight effect where everything seems to be speeded up. I once experienced this when out walking. I was getting very tired while trudging the last half mile when a car passed and splashed dirty water all over me from a puddle. I was furious and this led to a rise in adrenaline, which gave me the energy to almost sprint home. Cortisol increases blood sugar to give us the energy to fight or flee, it increases blood pressure and suppresses the immune system. This is one reason why stress can result in illness.

These two hormones are important because they help us to deal with the problem that is bothering us at the time. After the situation has ended, the levels of these hormones should return to normal. The problem is that sometimes they don't, and we might live with chronically high levels of cortisol and adrenaline for long periods. This can damage our health. Cortisol should be highest in the morning and become less as the day goes on. It should be lowest at night so that we are able to relax and sleep. Unfortunately, in some people, cortisol stays high into the evening and this keeps them awake.

The hormone dehydroepiandrosterone (DHEA) should be in balance with cortisol. It is a cortisol antagonist, which means that it dampens down the cortisol if we have too much. This means that the ratio between these two hormones is important and you can be tested for this (see below).

Cortisol and IBS

A study published in the medical journal *Biopsychosocial medicine* looked at female college students on a two-week course and found that those with IBS had a higher cortisol/DHEA ratio after awakening compared to those without IBS. The study concluded that 'the cortisol effect is dominant in individuals under prolonged stress'.[28] So trying to reduce this should help a lot.

Testing for high cortisol

A test for levels of cortisol, in which you collect saliva four times during the course of a day, can be done at home and sent to a laboratory for assessment.

Testing for cortisol/DHEA ratio

This is another valuable test because it looks at the balance of these two hormones. You take samples of your saliva four times a day, as in the previous test. As DHEA is a cortisol antagonist, this test will tell you if you have too much or too little of either. Tests can be carried out at Genova Diagnostics (www.gdx.net) or through a BANT nutritionist.

Lowering our stress levels

Since stress contributes to IBS and other digestive problems, it is important to try to relieve it as much as possible. I know that this is easier said than done. We don't choose to be stressed or to have the worries that we do. However, although lowering it might be difficult, it is not impossible.

Helping stress with nutrition

- Keep your blood sugar even by eating regular meals containing protein and complex carbohydrates, preferably in the form of vegetables. When blood sugar drops too low this causes more adrenaline to be produced.

- Eat a good breakfast on the lines described previously (protein and vegetables).

- Eat nutrient-dense foods by following the diet outlined in this book and eat natural, whole, unprocessed real foods (see Chapter 7).

- Drink green tea, which contains a chemical called

L-theanine, an amino acid that helps produce alpha waves in the brain. These in turn help reduce the production of stress hormones. It is not high in caffeine but if you are concerned about this, you could try a decaffeinated version.

- Eat food high in magnesium such as green leafy vegetables. Magnesium is needed to balance calcium and we tend to eat quite a large amount of this.

- Calcium too is needed for relaxation. The greatest amount is found in sesame seeds but remember that vitamin D is needed for its absorption.

- The herb holy basil seems to be able to reduce cortisol.

- Try to eat few processed foods, no sugar and no hydrogenated fats.

Other ways to help stress

Food is important but it is not everything. There are other good ways to help us relax and relieve stress, discussed below.

Emotional freedom technique (EFT)

The emotional freedom technique is a method of tapping on acupressure points on the body to help relaxation and relieve stress. There are many good books and internet videos that show you how to do this. It is very simple but can be effective.

Cognitive behavioural therapy (CBT)

Are you a real worrier? Are your thoughts controlling you instead of you controlling them? If so, you might like to try CBT. This type of therapy has proved to be very useful in the treatment of stress, anxiety and other disorders, and is usually short term. It works by helping us to stop thinking the worst about things and helps us to see things in a more positive light.

You may have become used to thinking in a way that is unhelpful to you and that affects your stress levels. For example, if a friend seems to ignore you in the street you might see this as a deliberate slight. This could lead you to feel upset, causing stomach pains, etc. However, it might just be that the friend was distracted or was worrying about something in their own life. If you see the situation in a different way, you will not be upset and the physical symptoms will not occur.

In one study published in the *European Journal of Gastroenterology Hepatology*, ninety female nursing students diagnosed with IBS were divided at random into two groups. One group was given eight weeks of CBT, while the other group was just given general information on IBS. After eight, sixteen and twenty-four weeks the severity of their bowel symptoms, dysfunctional attitude and IBS quality of life were assessed. In the CBT group the overall quality of life improved and the study concluded that CBT 'proved to be an effective intervention' in the IBS patients.[29]

Yoga

This is a very good way of helping stress and promoting relaxation. It is gentle and many people enjoy it very much, and it can also help IBS. Even children can benefit from yoga. A pilot study published in the journal *Complementary Therapies in Medicine* found that 'yoga exercises are effective for children . . . resulting in significant reduction of pain intensity and frequency, especially in children of 8-11 years old'.[30]

Listening to music

Do you love music? I do hope so because music not only gives us pleasure but relaxes us too. A review of twenty-two different studies published in the *Journal of Music Therapy* found that music with other relaxation techniques significantly reduced stress arousal.[31] An even more interesting finding was that music alone was able to do the same thing.

Mindfulness

This form of stress reduction has become very popular and research shows that it can help IBS. Mindfulness is a way of thinking that keeps us focused on the present. So often, when we are doing something our minds are not fully focused on what we are doing. We are thinking of what has happened in the past, worrying about what might happen in the future or going over and over things that have upset us. Mindfulness shows us how to stay in the present, pay attention to what we are actually doing and attend to that with our whole mind. For example, when children are playing, they give their full attention to what they are doing at the time. They are not ruminating about the past or thinking about what they might do tomorrow but, rather, they are fully focused on what has been called 'the now'.

Mindfulness and IBS

There is evidence that this can help IBS. A study published in the *American Journal of Gastroenterology* found that women who had undergone training in mindfulness did better than those who did not.[32] This was a randomized controlled trial where the women were assigned to either a group having mindfulness training or to a support group. Women in the mindfulness group 'showed greater reductions in IBS symptom severity after training and at 3-month follow up relative to the support group'. The study concluded that mindfulness training had a 'substantial therapeutic effect on bowel symptom severity'. The fact that it was a randomized controlled trial rather than an observation adds credibility to the study.

Meditation

Other forms of meditation, along with tapes that use visualization, are also very helpful in relieving the symptoms of stress. Of all types of meditation, some argue that transcendental meditation is the best. This can be expensive to learn but, if you cannot afford it, other types can be effective.

Exercise

We are always being told that we should exercise more. Those of us who are not naturally athletic, including me, might find this a bit challenging. However, we should all try to do exercise regularly because it is one of the best ways to lower stress hormones. High levels of adrenaline and cortisol are designed to enable us to take action against our problems. This helps us to fight or flee a bad situation, but after the stressor has gone, we need to calm down and relax again. The problem is that often this relaxation never really happens and we keep on feeling stressed, with raised cortisol and adrenaline staying around for long periods. Exercise uses up these stress hormones, allowing us to relax.

Exercise and IBS

Exercise does not just relieve stress as research has shown that it can help IBS in other ways. One study published in the *American Journal of Gastroenterology* concluded that, 'Increased physical activity improves GI symptoms in IBS. Physically active patients with IBS will face less symptom deterioration compared with physically inactive patients. Physical activity should be used as a primary treatment modality in IBS.'[33] This was a good study because it involved a randomized controlled trial in which patients were divided into two groups, with only one group exercising.

Some of us might not be very keen on exercise if we are not used to it, but it does not have to be difficult or unpleasant.

I think that it is important for people to find something they enjoy. It might be dancing, for example, and lately ballroom and Latin dancing have become very popular and many say that it makes them feel that they are walking on air. Happily, recent research has found that any type of exercise is valuable, even the exercise we naturally get when shopping, going about our daily lives and doing housework such as ironing, cleaning and gardening. If you like walking around shops, just enjoy it. You do not need to do all the day's exercise at once. Going out for a few walks throughout the day is just as beneficial. Swimming is good for people who find walking difficult or who have painful joints. It all counts as useful exercise and can add up to quite a lot over the whole day.

In a nutshell

- Eating under stress affects digestion.

- Evidence suggests that IBS is a stress-sensitive disorder.

- Try to relax while eating, and eat calmly and slowly at the table.

- To help stress eat meals (including breakfast) of protein and vegetables to keep blood sugar balanced.

- To reduce the effects of stress overall try techniques like yoga, meditation, mindfulness and cognitive behavioural therapy.

- Regular exercise is a good way to help stress. Try to do something you enjoy!

Chapter 11

SLEEP AND IBS

Do you sleep well? I hope so because a good night's sleep is so important for all aspects of our health, and this means our digestion too. On the other hand, do you wake up at all hours through the night or too early in the morning and find it hard to get back to sleep? Many of us do. Insomnia is extremely common, so much so that it is almost an epidemic. It can be horrible tossing and turning, getting up, trying to get back to sleep again, worrying about not sleeping. Then when you do drop off, it's time to get up. It can all be very debilitating.

Studies have shown that there is a connection between IBS and not sleeping well. In fact, one study published in the *Journal of Clinical Sleep Medicine* looked at how women with IBS felt bad after a poor night's sleep.[34] Those who reported poor sleep seemed to have a worsening of their symptoms the next day. It is therefore a good idea to try to improve your sleep as much as possible if you are not already sleeping well. I realize that this is often easier said than done but overleaf are some good ideas that may help.

How to improve sleep with nutrition

Improving your diet overall and eating the foods suggested in this book (see Chapter 7) should go a long way towards helping you sleep well. However, there are other things that you can do in addition to ensure a good night's sleep.

- *Avoid stimulants*: most of us now know that tea and coffee can keep us awake. If you think this is a problem for you, maybe just drink earlier on in the day. Chocolate, tobacco and alcohol can also affect sleep, although some people are more sensitive to these than others. Some people think that alcohol helps them sleep, but the sleep is not a proper refreshing sleep.

- *Increase foods that make serotonin*: this is converted to melatonin, which we need for sleep. It comes from an amino acid called tryptophan in protein foods. So eat turkey, chicken, cottage cheese (if not dairy intolerant) and enough protein foods throughout the day.

- *Eat half a banana* before bed as these also contain tryptophan.

- *Increase calcium and magnesium*: we looked at calcium and magnesium with regard to stress (see Chapter 10) but these are also needed for sleep. You need to make sure that you are getting enough of these from your diet. Foods high in calcium tend to be dairy products, which can be a problem if you cannot tolerate them so see the box overleaf for non-dairy, calcium-rich foods.

- *Try the supplement 5-Hydroxytryptophan (5HTP)*: this is sold in health-food shops and can help sleep.

Non-dairy calcium-rich foods	
Sesame seeds	Sunflower seeds
Sardines	Cabbage
Almonds	Broccoli
Trout	Chickpeas
Brazil nuts	Kale
Kelp	Soya beans
Goat's milk	

As mentioned in Chapter 8, many people have diets very high in calcium and low in magnesium. This is a problem because magnesium is needed in order to use the calcium. If it cannot be metabolized properly, it can be deposited in our soft tissue.

It is easy to get too much calcium in relation to magnesium because there are so many calcium-rich foods (cheeses, yogurts, etc.) on the market but foods that are high in magnesium are not as popular. Many do not like magnesium-rich green leafy vegetables or forget about nuts and seeds. Try adding magnesium-rich foods (see opposite) to your diet or take supplements.

Magnesium-rich foods	
Almonds	Fresh peas
Cashew nuts	Bananas
Wheatgerm	Celery
Brazil nuts	Millet
Parsley	Green leafy vegetables

Although nuts are high in magnesium it might be better to leave these out (or grind them) until your IBS is better as they can be very difficult to digest.

Magnesium baths

If you add some magnesium salts to your bath, you can absorb some magnesium through your skin. It is a little like the baths that people take in highly mineralized water at spas.

The magic of melatonin

We have seen, therefore, that a good night's sleep is very important for those with IBS because it is now known that this can affect our digestive system. One aspect of sleep, or at least lying in the dark, that is particularly important is the production of melatonin. It is known that melatonin is involved in the regulation of gastrointestinal motility and sensation. It can reduce abdominal pain and help deal with IBS symptoms.

Sleep in the dark

Melatonin is important and it can be increased with medication. If you do not want to take this, you need not worry because recent research has now shown that melatonin can now be increased naturally. Melatonin is produced when we are in the dark and stops being made when we are in the light. (At night, if we put the light on to visit the toilet, our levels of melatonin plummet.) One way that we can increase it is by sleeping in a completely darkened room. Fortunately for people who have trouble sleeping, the exciting research proves that we do not actually need to be asleep to produce melatonin. We now know that our production of it is completely regulated by light/darkness and not by sleeping.

We are meant to sleep when the sun goes down and rise when it gets light. However, in the modern world we have artificial light at night, light from computers and light in our bedrooms from clock radios and other devices. Even with our eyes closed, they will still perceive the light. This is a good reason to have curtains that block out the light. The silk eye-masks they give you on airlines are also effective. It is also a good idea to keep our house lights low after dark as bright, artificial light can prevent melatonin from reaching its highest point. Working on a computer late at night is also not a good idea. Strangely enough, the opposite effect happens during the day. You need to get some light then in order to sleep well at night.

I was amazed and delighted when I read the words of Professor Steven Hill from Tulane University: 'Our levels of melatonin are not determined by sleep, as many people think. It is the darkness that is important. During the night, if you sleep in a brightly lit room, your melatonin levels may be inhibited; however if you are in the dark but cannot sleep, your melatonin levels will rise normally.'[35]

That is great news for those who are not sleeping well. You can take heart that if you are in a darkened room, your melatonin levels can still be good, even if you are awake.

Melatonin and IBS

An interesting thing about melatonin is that it seems to be involved in digestion and in particular it is important for IBS. One study found that IBS scores in patients were much improved after taking melatonin. This was a randomized controlled trial in which some patients were given the melatonin and others a placebo or dummy pill. The results showed that those taking the melatonin experienced greater improvement than those on the placebo. The report concluded that, 'melatonin is a promising therapeutic agent for IBS'.[36] This was just one study but a review of seventeen non-clinical studies and eight clinical trials found that IBS patients tended to be low in melatonin and that when given melatonin they experienced a decrease in abdominal pain and improved overall IBS symptom scores.[37] Giving melatonin to sufferers resulted in decreased abdominal pain and overall improvement in other symptoms. The study concluded that, 'the results of seventeen non-clinical studies showed anxiolytic [anxiety-preventative], anti-inflammatory, anti-oxidative and motility regulatory effects of melatonin on the GI tract'.

While it is possible to get supplements of melatonin, I think it is better to do our best to increase this more naturally, such as sleeping in a darkened room and eating the right foods.

Food for melatonin production

Although we need darkness to make melatonin, we also need the nutrients from which it is made. We need the amino acid tryptophan, which comes from food, to make serotonin, which in turn makes melatonin. Foods high in tryptophan are:

- Turkey and chicken – do you fall asleep after a Christmas dinner?

- Eggs.

- Sesame seeds and various nuts (chew very well or grind).

- Protein foods in general, so be careful about getting enough if you are a vegetarian. Protein is needed throughout the day so that we can make serotonin at night.

- Camomile tea is relaxing.
- Half a banana can sometimes help.

Test for melatonin

This can be done via a saliva test, which is easy to do and is also very accurate. There are private laboratories that can do this for you.

Waking in the middle of the night

Do you find that you wake up in the middle of the night and can't get back to sleep again for a long time? This can be very annoying and upsetting. We now know that it can be caused by your blood sugar dropping too low. When this happens, adrenaline is released into the bloodstream and this in turn keeps us awake. In order to stop this happening you need to eat some protein and complex carbohydrates in the evening, which should help keep your blood sugar stable for longer. High carbohydrate foods like biscuits, cakes and bread will do the opposite. They will cause a sharp rise in blood sugar when you eat them but this is followed by a drop a few hours later.

If you wake during the night, a small piece of protein such as leftover chicken and half a small banana should help you get back to sleep.

In a nutshell

- IBS and poor sleep are related.

- Melatonin is important both for sleep and for preventing IBS.

- Many IBS sufferers are low in melatonin.

- Melatonin is produced in the dark and stops being produced when our eyes experience light.

- Eating the best diet with enough protein and minerals such as calcium and magnesium is needed for sleep.

- Some foods contain tryptophan, which is needed to make serotonin, which converts to melatonin.

- Stress management is also important (see Chapter 10).

SUMMARY

Now we have come to the end of the programme and I hope that you have discovered the cause of your problems. It may take some time and effort to make it work for you but, if you persevere, it should. We have gone through the causes of most symptoms and, if you have discovered these and dealt with them, you should now feel much better.

We looked at what we should not have in our digestive tract and these are:

- small intestinal bacterial overgrowth (SIBO);
- wheat;
- candida overgrowth;
- parasites.

We looked at what we should have:

- enough fibre;
- enough stomach acid;
- enough digestive enzymes;
- the best and most nutritious foods.

Then we added back:

- probiotics – beneficial bacteria to replenish our stores;
- prebiotics – to feed the probiotics.

Finally, we attempted to:

- heal any inflammation and leaky gut with foods and supplements.

Side benefits of the plan

Having done all that, you should end up with better digestion and much more, assuming that you are now eating good foods. If we are digesting our food properly, we should be protected from all kinds of other illnesses as many of them come from not absorbing the nutrients and minerals in food. In fact, it is amazing how many problems good digestion can help protect you from or alleviate. Here are just a few examples:

- *Osteoporosis*: about seventeen different nutrients are needed to make bone but just eating foods rich in these is not enough to prevent osteoporosis. We also need good digestive health to make sure that we are absorbing the nutrients properly.

- *Anaemia*: in order to prevent this, we need to be able to absorb iron and vitamin B12 properly. Good levels of stomach acid are required for this.

- *Skin health, fertility and good immunity*: all of these, as well as the manufacture of stomach acid, require good levels of zinc.

- *Leaky gut*: if we do not have a leaky gut we are less at risk of autoimmune diseases such as thyroiditis, multiple sclerosis, scleroderma and a whole host of others.

- *Cancer, heart disease, type 2 diabetes*: if we can properly absorb vitamins, minerals, the right fats and phytochemicals, we will be more protected from these illnesses.

- In fact, a well-functioning digestive system is paramount for all aspects of good health.

Lastly, I hope that you will all enjoy eating for health and that it will be a pleasure and not a chore. Food is there to be enjoyed and there is no need to use complicated recipes. Simple ways of cooking are just as good.

I wish you all happy eating and the very best of health!

NOTES

Chapter 3

1. I. Moraru et al., 'Small intestinal bacterial overgrowth is associated to symptoms in irritable bowel syndrome: evidence from a multicentre study in Romania', *Romanian Journal of Internal Medicine*, 52: 3 (2014), 143–50.

2. E. Lipski, *Digestive Wellness* (New York: McGraw-Hill, 2012).

3. D. Perlmutter, *Grain Brain* (London: Yellow Kite, 2014).

4. E. F. Verdu, 'Can gluten contribute to irritable bowel syndrome?', *American Journal of Gastroenterology*, 106: 3 (March 2011), 516–18.

5. W. Davis, *Wheat Belly* (New York: Rodale, 2011).

6. C. Zioudrou et al., 'Opiod peptides derived from food proteins: the exorphins', *Journal of Biological Chemistry*, 254: 7 (April 1979), 2446–9.

7. S. Bijan et al., 'Non-celiac gluten sensitivity has narrowed the spectrum of irritable bowel syndrome: a double-blind randomized placebo-controlled trial', *Nutrients*, 7: 6 (June 2015), 4542–54.

8. W. Davis, *Wheat Belly* (New York: Rodale, 2011).

9. D. Stark, 'Irritable bowel syndrome: a review on the role of intestinal protozoa and the importance of their detection and diagnosis', *International Journal of Parasitology*, 37: 1 (2007), 11–20.

10. W. Crook, *The Yeast Connection* (New York: Random House, 1988).

Chapter 5

11. T. Didari et al., 'Effectiveness of probiotics in irritable bowel syndrome: updated systematic review with meta-analysis', *World Journal of Gastroenterology*, 21: 10 (14 March 2015), 3072–84.

12. C. Choi et al., 'A randomized, double-blind, placebo-controlled multi-center trial of *Saccharomyces boulardii* in irritable bowel syndrome: effect on quality of life', *Journal of Clinical Gastroenterology*, 45; 8 (September 2011), 679–83.

13. S. Hertzler, 'Kefir improves lactose digestion and tolerance in adults

with lactose maldigestion', *Journal of the American Dietetic Association*, 103: 5 (May 2003), 582–7.

Chapter 6

14. S. Rogers, *No More Heartburn: Stop the Pain in 30 Days – Naturally! The Safe, Effective Way to Prevent and Heal Chronic Gastrointestinal Disorders* (New York: Kensington Publishing Corporation, 2000).

15. S. P. Dunlop *et al.*, 'Abnormal intestinal permeability in subgroups of diarrhoea-predominant irritable bowel syndromes', *American Journal of Gastroenterology*, 101: 6 (June 2006), 1288–94.

16. Rogers, *No More Heartburn*.

17. Rogers, *No More Heartburn*.

18. R. Bundy *et al.*, 'Turmeric extract may improve irritable bowel syndrome symptomology in otherwise healthy adults: a pilot study', *Journal of Alternative and Complementary Medicine*, 10: 6 (December 2004), 1015–18.

Chapter 7

19. I. Chirila *et al.*, 'Diet and irritable bowel syndrome', *Journal of Gastrointestinal Liver Diseases*, 21: 4 (December 2012), 357–62.

20. S. Sonja *et al.*, 'Zinc and gastrointestinal disease', *World Journal of Gastrointestinal Pathophysiology*, 5: 4 (15 November 2014), 496–513.

21. T. Solakivi *et al.*, 'Serum fatty acid profile in subjects with irritable bowel syndrome', *Scandinavian Journal of Gastroenterology*, 46: 3 (March 2011), 299–303.

22. Y. Khayyat *et al.*, 'Vitamin D deficiency in patients with irritable bowel syndrome: does it exist?', *Oman Medical Journal*, 30: 2 (March 2015), 115–18.

Chapter 8

23. K. Murakami *et al.*, 'Association between dietary fiber, water and magnesium intake and functional constipation among young Japanese women', *European Journal of Clinical Nutrition*, 61: 5 (May 2007), 616–22.

24. I. Turan *et al.*, 'Effects of a kefir supplement on symptoms, colonic transit, and bowel satisfaction score in patients with chronic constipation: a pilot study', *Turkish Journal of Gastroenterology*, 25: 6 (December 2014), 650–56.

25. Rogers, *No More Heartburn*.

Chapter 10

26. M. Lin Chang, 'The role of stress on physiological responses and clinical symptoms in irritable bowel syndrome', *Gastroenterology*, 140: 3 (March 2011), 761–5.

27. Q. Hong-Yan *et al.*, 'Impact of psychological stress on irritable bowel syndrome', *World Journal of Gastroenterology*, 20: 39 (21 October 2014), 14126–31.

28. N. Sugaya *et al.*, 'Effect of prolonged stress on the adrenal hormones of individuals with irritable bowel syndrome', *Biopsychosocial Medicine*, 9: 1 (23 January 2015), 4.

29. A. L. Jang *et al.*, 'The effects of cognitive behavioural therapy in female nursing students with irritable bowel syndrome: a randomized trial', *European Journal of Gastroenterology Hepatology*, 26: 8 (August 2014): 918–26.

30. M. Brands *et al.*, 'A pilot study of yoga treatment in children with functional abdominal pain and irritable bowel syndrome', *Complementary Therapies in Medicine*, 19: 3 (June 2011), 109–14.

31. C. L. Pelletier, 'The effect of music on decreasing arousal due to stress: a meta-analysis', *Journal of Music Therapy*, 41: 3 (Fall 2004): 192–214.

32. S. Gaylord *et al.*, 'Mindfulness training reduces the severity of irritable bowel syndrome in women: results of a randomized controlled trial', *American Journal of Gastroenterology*, 106: 9 (September 2011), 1678–88.

33. E. Johannesson *et al.*, 'Physical activity improves symptoms in irritable bowel syndrome: a randomized controlled trial', *American Journal of Gastroenterology*, 106: 5 (May 2011), 915–22.

Chapter 11

34. D. Buchanan *et al.*, 'Sleep measures predict next-day symptoms in women with irritable bowel syndrome', *Journal of Clinical Sleep Medicine*, 10: 9 (15 September 2014), 1003–9.

35. R. Dauchy *et al.*, 'Circadian and melatonin disruption by exposure to light at night drives intrinsic resistance to tamoxifen therapy in breast cancer', *Cancer Research*, 74: 15 (2014), 1–12.

36. W. Lu *et al.*, 'Melatonin improves bowel symptoms in female patients with irritable bowel syndrome: a double-blind placebo-controlled study', *Ailment Pharmacological Therapy*, 22: 10 (15 November 2005), 927–34.

37. S. Mozaffari *et al.*, 'Implications of melatonin therapy in irritable bowel syndrome: a systematic review', *Current Pharmacological Design*, 16: 33 (November 2010), 3646–55.

INDEX

177

Index